Clinician's Manual on
Axial Spondyloarthritis

Clinician's Manual on Axial Spondyloarthritis

Joachim Sieper
Charité University Hospital
Campus Benjamin Franklin
Berlin
Germany

Jürgen Braun
Rheumatology Center
Ruhrgebiet St Josefs Hospital
Herne
Germany

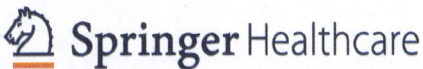

Published by Springer Healthcare Ltd, 236 Gray's Inn Road, London, WC1X 8HB, UK.

www.springerhealthcare.com

British Library Cataloguing-in-Publication Data.

A catalogue record for this book is available from the British Library.

ISBN 978-1-907673-84-9

Project editor: Tess Salazar
Production: Dorothy Davis
Printed in Great Britain by Latimer Trend

Contents

Authors' biographies

Joachim Sieper, MD, is a Consultant and Head of Rheumatology at the Charité University Hospital, Campus Benjamin Franklin in Berlin, Germany. After receiving his medical degree in 1978 from Free University, in Berlin, Germany, he underwent his training in internal medicine in the Department of Cardiology at the Rudolf–Virchow clinic in Berlin, Germany. He continued his training in internal medicine and rheumatology at the University Hospital Benjamin Franklin, in Berlin, Germany. During this time he had a number of fellowships abroad including 8 weeks at The London Lupus Clinic, Hammersmith Hospital, in London, UK, led by Professor Graham Hughes. He also spent over a year at the Rheumatology Unit of Guy's Hospital, in London, UK, led by Professor G Panayi. In 1998 he became Professor of Medicine at Free University and that same year he was also appointed Deputy Head of the Department of Internal Medicine at the same institution. In 2000 he became Head of Rheumatology at Free University.

Professor Sieper is also a prolific researcher and writer. He has been an investigator since 1989, and a principal investigator since 1993 on several placebo-controlled randomized trials, which have been published internationally. He has authored and contributed to over 300 journal papers.

He is a member of numerous societies including the German Society of Rheumatology and the American College of Rheumatology.

He has also been the recipient of many awards and honors for excellence in rheumatology, including the Carol-Nachman award for rheumatology in 2000 and the European League Against Rheumatism (EULAR) award in 2003.

Jürgen Braun, MD, is Medical Director of the Rheumatology Medical Centre, Ruhrgebiet in Herne, Germany, and is a lecturer at the Ruhr University in Bochum, Germany. He is also an honorary Professor in Rheumatology at the Charité Medical School in Berlin, Germany.

He received his doctor of medicine degree in 1987 at the Free University, Berlin, Germany, and went on to become certified as a specialist in rheumatology, internal medicine, laboratory medicine, physical therapy, and sports medicine. In 2000, he became Professor of Rheumatology at the Free University, Berlin. The following year he became Medical Director of the Rheumatology Medical Centre, Ruhrgebiet in Herne, one of the major hospitals in Germany specialized in the management of patients with rheumatic diseases, a position he still holds.

Professor Braun has been an invited speaker at a number of universities and institutions including the National Institutes of Health, the American College of Rheumatology, the European League Against Rheumatism (EULAR), and the Asia Pacific League of Associations for Rheumatology. He has also been invited to speak about his research at the national meetings of the British, Irish, Indian, Scandinavian, Danish, Dutch, Belgian, Italian, Spanish, Greek, Turkish, Moroccan, Russian, Chinese, and German Society of Rheumatology. In 2004, he was appointed as the inaugural Robert Inman lecturer at the University of Toronto, Canada.

Professor Braun has been the recipient of several prestigious awards, including the Ankylosing Spondylitis Patients Association Award in 1996, the Tosse-Research Award in Pediatric Rheumatology in 1998, the Carol-Nachman Research Award in 2000, and the EULAR prize in 2003.

As one of the leading specialists in the field of the spondyloarthritides, Professor Braun has published more than 300 papers on different aspects of this subject. He is a member of the Steering Committee of the Assessments in Ankylosing Spondylitis Working group and the Group for Research and Assessment of Psoriasis and Psoriatic Arthritis.

Acknowledgements

Our thanks go to our colleagues in the Assessment in SpondyloArthritis international Society (ASAS) for their permission to reproduce Figures 3.8, 4.3, 4.4, 4.5, 5.1, 6.8, and 6.19 in this manual.

Abbreviations

AS	ankylosing spondylitis
ASAS	Assessment in SpondyloArthritis international Society
ASDAS	Ankylosing Spondylitis Disease Activity Score
axSpA	axial spondyloarthritis
BASDAI	Bath Ankylosing Spondylitis Disease Activity Index
BASMI	Bath Ankylosing Spondylitis Metrology Index
BASFI	Bath Ankylosing Spondylitis Functional Index
CRP	C-reactive protein
CT	computed tomography
DISH	diffuse idiopathic skeletal hyperostosis
DMARD	disease-modifying antirheumatic drug
ESR	erythrocyte sedimentation rate
ESSG	European Spondyloarthropathy Study Group
EULAR	European League Against Rheumatism
HLA	human leukocyte antigen
IBD	inflammatory bowel disease
IBP	inflammatory back pain
IL	interleukin
LR	likelihood ratio
MASES	Maastricht Ankylosing Spondylitis Enthesitis Score
MRI	magnetic resonance imaging
NRS	numerical rating scale
nr-axSpA	nonradiographic axial spondyloarthritis
NSAID	nonsteroidal anti-inflammatory drug
SI	sacroiliac
SpA	spondyloarthritis
STIR	short tau inversion recovery
TB	tuberculosis
Th-17	T-helper cell 17
TNF	tumor necrosis factor
VAS	visual analogue scale

Chapter 1

Introduction

The term axial spondyloarthritis (axSpA) covers both patients who already have radiographic changes in the sacroiliac joints (radiographic sacroiliitis, ankylosing spondylitis [AS]) and patients who do not have such changes; this subgroup is now called nonradiographic axSpA (nr-axSpA). AxSpA is more common in men than in women in case of established AS while in case of nr-axSpA there may even be a slight female predominance. AxSpA is a chronic inflammatory disease which, probably as a result of an autoimmune process, causes inflammation in sacroiliac joints, vertebrae, and adjacent joints. Patients also frequently have inflammation of entheses (insertions of tendons or ligaments into bone), the peripheral joints, and the eye. Next to axial inflammation the phenomenon of new bone formation is pathognomonic for axSpA and especially AS. In severe cases fusion of vertebral bodies to the so-called bamboo spine is observed. Both inflammation and new bone formation may significantly impact patients' mobility and function. In AS, other organs, such as heart valves, kidneys, and lungs, are only rarely affected. The onset of symptoms – notably back pain and stiffness – occurs often already in adolescence or early adulthood. To date, the disease has no cure, but medical and physical therapy may improve pain, inflammation, and other symptoms considerably; indeed, even remission has now become a realistic goal. A major breakthrough in the treatment of this disease, next to the efficacy of nonsteroidal anti-inflammatory drugs (NSAID), was the demonstration of the partly impressive efficacy of tumor necrosis factor (TNF)-blocking agents [1].

J. Sieper and J. Braun, *Clinician's Manual on Axial Spondyloarthritis*,
DOI: 10.1007/978-1-907673-85-6_1, © Springer Healthcare 2014

The diagnosis of axSpA is often delayed as symptoms can be confused with other more common, but usually less serious disorders, such as chronic low back pain, which is a frequent complaint that gives reason to visits of general practitioners, orthopedists, and physiatrists. Furthermore, typical radiological changes of the sacroiliac joints may become visible only after some time, often years of ongoing inflammation. However, 20–30% of patients with axSpA develop structural changes already in the first two years of disease. Therefore, the term "axial spondyloarthritis" should be used now, which covers both patients with AS and those with nonradiographic sacroiliitis. Early diagnosis and intervention can, however, minimize or even prevent years of pain and disability.

In the face of these challenges, the *Clinician's Manual on Axial Spondyloarthritis* provides a concise, clinically focused overview of the manifestations, diagnosis, and management of this potentially debilitating condition. The AS subgroup will often be discussed first in this manual because more data are available here, followed by presenting data on nr-axSpA and/or axSpA in total. For some sections, only AS data are available at present.

A historical perspective

Studies of Egyptian mummies indicate that the disease now known as AS has afflicted humankind since antiquity. The first historical description of AS appeared in the literature in 1559 when Realdo Colombo provided an anatomical description of two skeletons with abnormalities typical of AS. More than 100 years later, the Irish doctor Bernard Connor described a bony fusion of spine and sacroiliac joints of a human skeleton. Despite several descriptions of conditions resembling AS later on, the reports of Bechterew in Russia (1893), Strümpell in Germany (1897), and Marie in France (1898) are often cited as the first descriptions of AS. Around 1900 the terms "Bechterew's disease", used preferentially in German-speaking countries and Russia, and "ankylosing spondylitis" were introduced.

At this time a diagnosis could be made only when a patient with AS had already developed the typical posture (see Figure 1.1A) that results from an advanced ankylosis of the spine or post mortem [2]. It was not until the 1930s that roentgenology was applied to AS, and it became evident from these studies that, in about 95% of cases, the sacroiliac joint is affected in AS (Figure 1.1B) [2]. These findings are the basis for the prominent role of radiographic sacroiliitis in the currently used diagnostic and classification criteria for AS, such as the 1984 modified New York criteria [3]. However, there was already some evidence (both clinically and from scintigraphy) that patients may have symptoms caused by inflammation many years before structural damage becomes visible on radiographs. The presence of an inflammatory nonradiographic stage early in the course of the disease became much clearer when magnetic resonance imaging (MRI) was used in AS in the 1990s (Figure 1.1C) [2]. Consequently, acute inflammatory sacroiliitis shown by MRI has become part of the new classification criteria for axSpA.

Historical aspects of ankylosing spondylitis

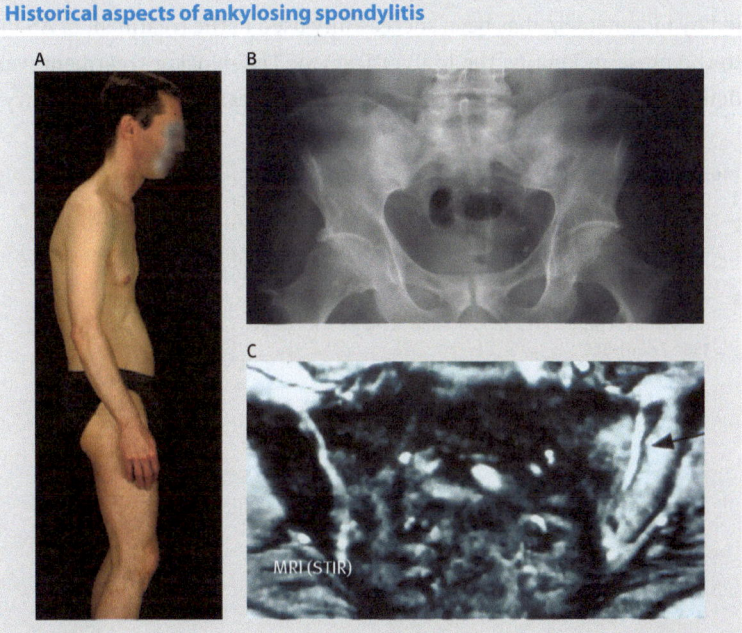

Figure 1.1 Historical aspects of ankylosing spondylitis. A, in the 1900s, a diagnosis could only be made when the patient exhibited the typical posture associated with AS; **B,** a radiograph showing bilateral sacroiliitis; roentgenology began to be applied to AS in the 1930s; **C,** a MRI showing a patient with acute sacroiliitis; the use of MRI in the early 1990s helped to identify the presence of an inflammatory nonradiographic stage early in the course of AS. AS, ankylosing spondylitis; STIR, short tau inversion recovery. Reproduced with permission from © John Wiley and Sons 2013, Braun et al [2]. All Rights Reserved.

Starting in the 1920s, radiation treatment was used for patients with AS to treat spinal pain and had good results, such as improvement of the symptoms. However, this therapy was abandoned because of the serious long-term side effects of such treatment, such as leukemia and other malignancies. Although treatment with salicylates has been used for the treatment of inflammatory rheumatic diseases since about 1900, this drug was not effective in AS. Phenylbutazone was introduced into clinical practice in 1949 and became the first drug to which the term "nonsteroidal anti-inflammatory drug" was applied. It has been highly effective for the treatment of AS with control of pain and inflammation. Yet its use has been restricted to only short-term treatment of AS because of potentially serious side effects, notably aplastic anemia and hepatic injury. Subsequently, since around 1965, a second generation of NSAIDs, led by indometacin, has been successfully used in the treatment of AS up to the present. Finally, the high efficacy of TNF-blocker treatment was demonstrated in patients with AS in the first years of the new century.

References

1   Braun J, Sieper J. Ankylosing spondylitis. *Lancet*. 2007;369:1379-1390.
2   Braun J, Bollow M, Eggens U, König H, Distler A, Sieper J. Use of dynamic magnetic resonance imaging with fast imaging in the detection of early and advanced sacroiliitis in spondylarthropathy patients. *Arthritis Rheum*. 1994;37:1039-1045.
3   van der Linden S, Valkenburg HA, Cats A. Evaluation of diagnostic criteria for ankylosing spondylitis. A proposal for modification of the New York criteria. *Arthritis Rheum*. 1984;27:361-368.

Chapter 2

Overview of axial spondyloarthritis

The concept and classification of spondyloarthritis

The term "spondyloarthritis" (SpA) comprises ankylosing spondylitis (AS), reactive arthritis, arthritis/spondylitis associated with psoriasis, and arthritis/spondylitis associated with inflammatory bowel disease (IBD). There is considerable overlap between the single subsets (Figure 2.1).

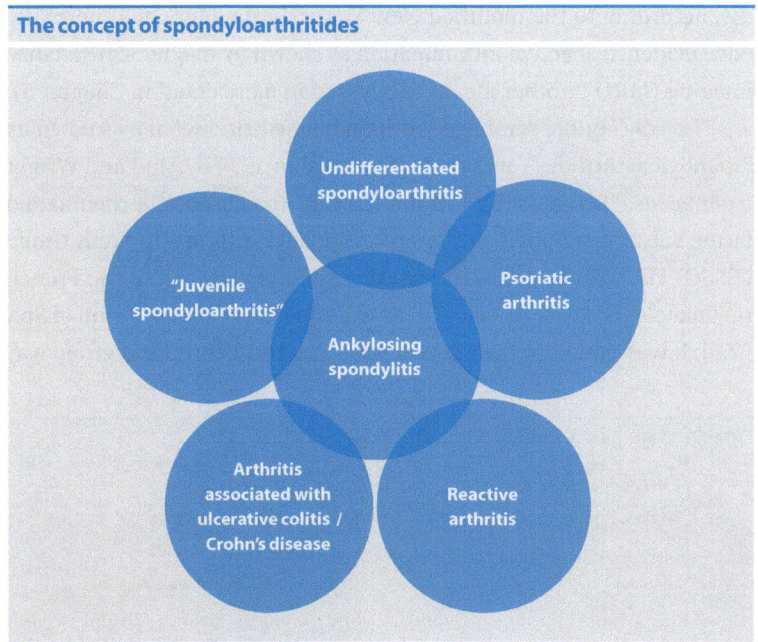

The concept of spondyloarthritides

Undifferentiated spondyloarthritis

"Juvenile spondyloarthritis"

Psoriatic arthritis

Ankylosing spondylitis

Arthritis associated with ulcerative colitis / Crohn's disease

Reactive arthritis

Figure 2.1 The concept of spondyloarthritides.

J. Sieper and J. Braun, *Clinician's Manual on Axial Spondyloarthritis*, DOI: 10.1007/978-1-907673-85-6_2, © Springer Healthcare 2014

The main link between each is the association with the human leukocyte antigen (HLA)-B27, the same pattern of peripheral joint involvement with an asymmetrical, often pauciarticular, arthritis, predominantly of the lower limbs, and the possible occurrence of sacroiliitis, spondylitis, enthesitis, dactylitis, and uveitis. All SpA subsets can evolve into AS, especially in those patients who are positive for HLA-B27. The SpA subsets can also be split into patients with predominantly axial and predominantly peripheral SpA (Figure 2.2), with an overlap between the two parts in about 20–40% of cases [1]. Through use of such a classification the presence or absence of evidence for a preceding gastrointestinal or urogenital infection, psoriasis or IBD is recorded but does not result in a different classification. The term "predominant axial SpA (axSpA)" covers patients with classic AS and those with nonradiographic axSpA (nr-axSpA) [1]. The latter group of patients would not have radiographic sacroiliitis, according to the modified New York criteria, but would normally have evidence of active inflammation as shown by magnetic resonance imaging (MRI) or other means (discussed in more detail in Chapter 5).

The concept of "seronegative spondyloarthritides", now known as "spondyloarthritides", was first introduced in 1974 by Moll and Wright from Leeds. "Seronegative" stands here for the absence of rheumatoid factor. Subsequently, both the European Spondyloarthropathy Study Group (ESSG) classification criteria and the Amor criteria (from the French rheumatologist Bernard Amor) tried to define the whole spectrum of SpA [2,3]. It was thanks to the ESSG criteria that in 1991 the SpA group was

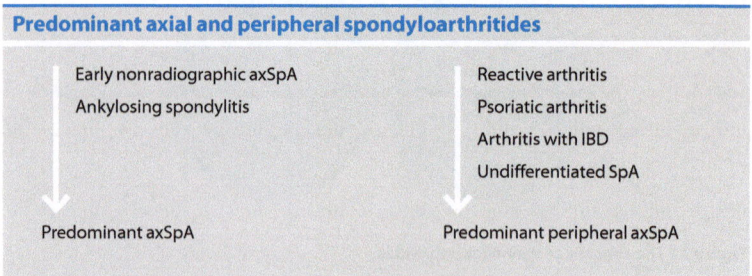

Predominant axial and peripheral spondyloarthritides

Early nonradiographic axSpA
Ankylosing spondylitis

Reactive arthritis
Psoriatic arthritis
Arthritis with IBD
Undifferentiated SpA

Predominant axSpA

Predominant peripheral axSpA

Figure 2.2 Predominant axial and peripheral spondyloarthritides. axSpA, axial spondyloarthritis; IBD, inflammatory bowel disease; SpA, spondyloarthritis. Adapted from Rudwaleit et al [1].

first split into predominantly axial and peripheral subsets. Figure 2.3 shows the current ESSG classification criteria for spondyloarthritis [2]. Most recently the Assessment in SpondyloArthritis international Society (ASAS) has proposed new classification criteria on axSpA, a term that is used throughout this book [4].

Epidemiology of axial spondyloarthritis

AxSpa is a disease that starts normally in the third decade of life, with about 80% of patients developing the first symptoms before the age of 30 and less than 5% of patients being older than 45 at the start of the disease. Up to 20% of patients are even younger than 20 years when they experience their first symptoms (Figure 2.4) [5]. Patients who are positive for HLA-B27 are about 10 years younger than HLA-B27-negative patients when the disease starts [6].

Men with AS are slightly more affected than are women, with a ratio of about 2:1, but women are equally affected compared to men in the nr-axSpA stage. Indeed, women generally develop chronic radiographic changes of the sacroiliac joints and the spine later than men, a possible explanation for the frequent underdiagnosis of AS in women in the past, resulting in a much higher male:female ratio than currently accepted [6].

European Spondyloarthropathy Study Group classification criteria for spondyloarthropathy		
Inflammatory back pain	**or**	**Synovitis**
		asymmetrical or
		predominantly in the lower limbs
plus one of the following:		
alternating buttock pain		
sacroiliitis		
heel pain (enthesitis)		
positive family history		
psoriasis		
Crohn's disease, ulcerative colitis		
urethritis/acute diarrhea in the preceding 4 weeks		

Figure 2.3 European Spondyloarthropathy Study Group classification criteria for spondyloarthropathy. Reproduced with permission from © John Wiley and Sons 2013, Dougados et al [2]. All Rights Reserved.

Age at first symptoms and at first diagnosis in patients with ankylosing spondylitis

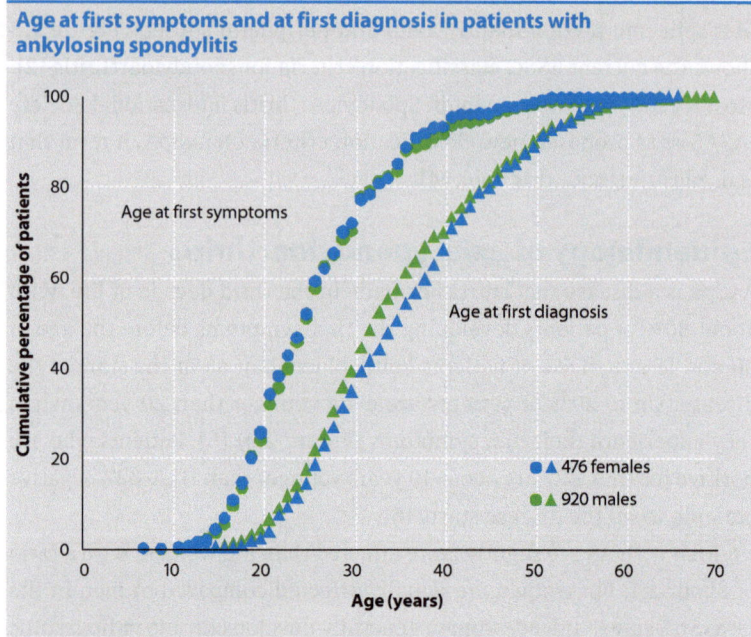

Figure 2.4 Age at first symptoms and at first diagnosis in patients with ankylosing spondylitis. Reproduced with permission from © Wolters Kluwer Health 2013, Feldtkeller et al [5]. All Rights Reserved.

There is a clear correlation between the prevalence of HLA-B27 and the prevalence of AS in a given population: the higher the HLA-B27 prevalence, the higher the AS prevalence. HLA-B27 is present throughout the world with a wide ethnic and geographical variation. It is most prevalent in northern countries and some tribes (Figure 2.5) [7–11]. Overall, estimations about the prevalence of AS are between 0.1% and 1.4%, with most of these data coming from Europe. In western and mid-Europe a prevalence of 0.3–0.5% for AS and of 1–2% for the whole SpA group is likely. Recent studies from France, the USA, and Lithuania indicate that SpA is at least as common as rheumatoid arthritis (Figure 2.6), which makes AS and SpA one of the most important chronic inflammatory rheumatic diseases [12–16]. A study from the USA reported an overall prevalence of axSpA of about 1% [17]. However, a major limitation of this study was the lack of information on sacroiliac joint imaging and HLA–B27 status of the patients.

Prevalence of ankylosing spondylitis

Country	AS prevalence	HLA-B27 prevalence
US [7]	1.0–1.5%	8%
The Netherlands [8]	0.1%	8%
Germany [9]	0.55%	9%
Norway [10]	1.1–1.4%	14%
Haida Indians [11]	6.1%	50%

Figure 2.5 Prevalence of ankylosing spondylitis. AS, ankylosing spondylitis; HLA, human leukocyte antigen. Adapted from Calin and Fries [7], van der Linden et al [8], Braun et al [9], Gran et al [10], Gofton et al [11].

Prevalence of spondyloarthritides and rheumatoid arthritis

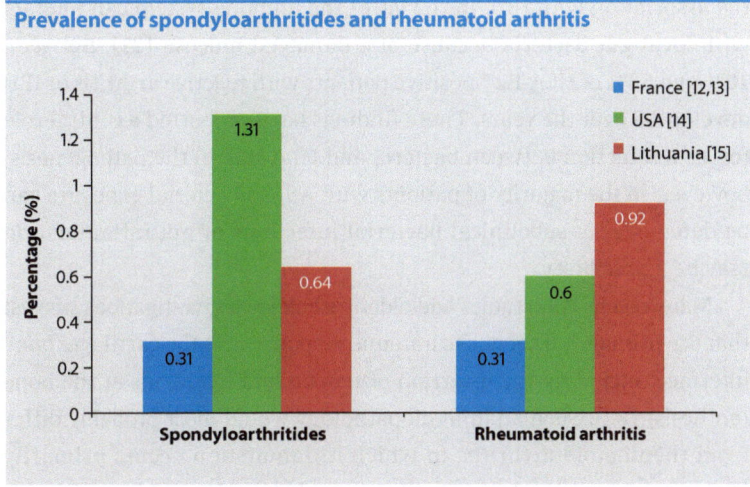

Figure 2.6 Prevalence of spondyloarthritides and rheumatoid arthritis. Adapted from Saraux et al [12], Guillemin et al [13], Adomaviciute et al [14], Helmick et al [15].

HLA-B27 is positive in 90–95% of patients with AS and in about 80–90% of patients with nr-axSpA. This percentage goes down to about 60% in patients with AS who also have psoriasis or IBD. In predominant peripheral SpA, less than 50% of patients are positive for HLA-B27.

Attempts have been made to estimate the ratio between patients with AS (radiographic axSpA) and nr-axSpA when a diagnosis of axSpA is first made by a rheumatologist. Nr-axSpA has been found in between 25% and 50% of patients with axSpA [18]. This proportion is higher when concentrating on patients with shorter symptom durations [19].

Etiopathogenesis of axial spondyloarthritis

A major breakthrough in the research on the pathogenesis of AS and related SpA was the reported strong association of the disease with HLA-B27 in 1973 [20]. However, intensive research over more than three decades has not clarified the functional role of the HLA-B27 molecule in the pathogenic process. The center of the discussion on the pathogenesis of SpA has long been the interaction between bacteria and HLA-B27, as a result of known triggering bacteria in reactive arthritis (after preceding bacterial infections of the urogenital or gastrointestinal tract) and the association with IBD; in the latter the immune system can interact with local gut bacteria because of a damaged mucosa [21]. Between 10% and 50% of HLA-B27-positive patients with reactive arthritis or IBD develop AS over the years. These findings have supported a central role for an interaction between bacteria and HLA-B27 in the pathogenesis; however, in the majority of patients with AS, no bacterial exposure can be detected, but subclinical bacterial infections or gut inflammation may be a possibility.

Many recent MRI studies and older pathological investigations suggest that the primary target of the immune response is at the cartilage/bone interface, including the insertion of tendon and ligaments at the bone (enthesis) [22]. Such an immunopathology would most probably differ from rheumatoid arthritis, in which inflammation occurs primarily in the synovium. We have recently provided further evidence for this hypothesis, showing that the presence of mononuclear cell infiltrates and osteoclasts depends on the presence of cartilage on the joint surface in patients with AS (Figure 2.7) [23,24]. However, there is currently no evidence that bacteria or bacterial antigens persist in the cartilage or close to the cartilage of spine and joints. Thus, there have been speculations that bacteria might trigger an autoimmune response against cartilage-derived antigens, such as proteoglycan or collagen, possibly mediated somehow through HLA-B27, although this hypothesis has not yet been proved. A third and necessary triggering component could be microtrauma(s) of cartilage/bone because weight-bearing parts of the skeleton are almost exclusively affected in axSpA. An elevated expression of the cytokines interleukin (IL)-17 [25] and IL-23 [26] have been found

Osteoclasts infiltrate at the bone–cartilage interface in patients with ankylosing spondylitis hip arthritis

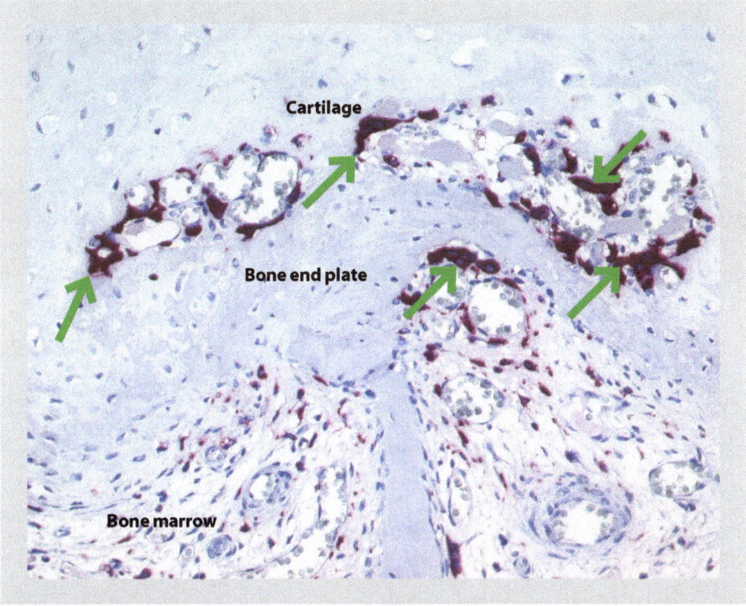

Figure 2.7 Osteoclasts infiltrate at the bone–cartilage interface in patients with ankylosing spondylitis hip arthritis. Osteoclasts are shown in green (arrows). Adapted from Appel and Sieper [24].

in the subchondral bone marrow of patients with AS and these cytokines have more recently gained much interest as potential treatment targets (see Chapter 6). Furthermore, IL-23 has been found to play a crucial role in the pathogenesis of enthesitis in an animal model with features resembling SpA [27].

In addition to inflammation, axSpA is also characterized by new bone formation, with the possible consequence of bone fusion, most frequently found in the axial skeleton in the form of syndesmophytes. For a long time there has been a question over how inflammation and new bone formation are coupled in AS, whether AS is a disease of excessive new bone formation or whether this is only part of a physiological repair mechanism. Figure 2.8 shows a likely sequence of events: first inflammation causes an osteitis, followed by erosive structural damage of bone and cartilage, which are filled with (fibrous) repair tissue, with a final step in

Proposed sequence of structural damage in ankylosing spondylitis

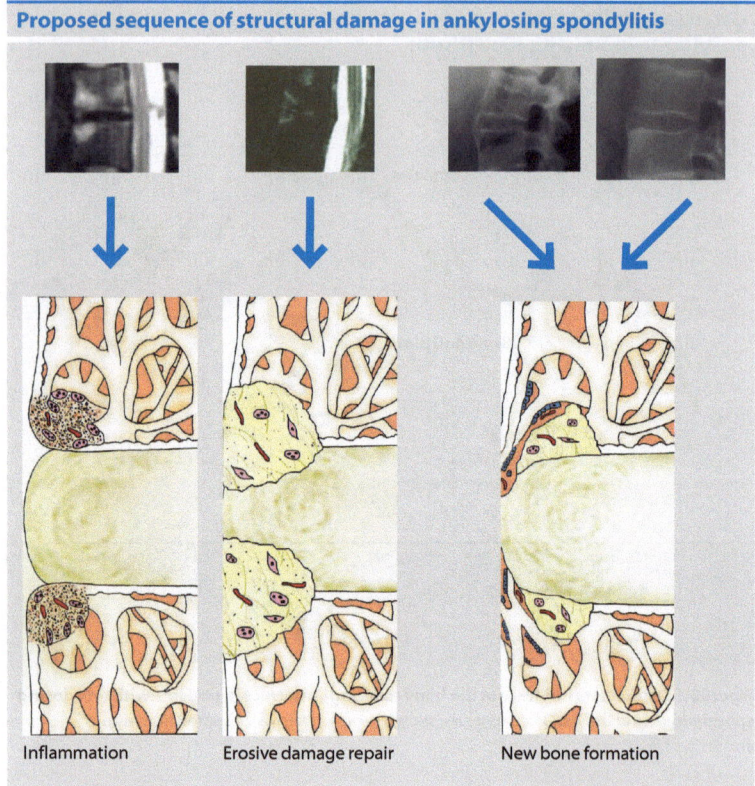

| Inflammation | Erosive damage repair | New bone formation |

Figure 2.8 Proposed sequence of structural damage in ankylosing spondylitis. Adapted from Appel and Sieper [24].

which this repair tissue is subsequently ossified [24]. If this is true, new bone formation would not occur without previous erosive damage from inflammation [24,28,29]. Interestingly, the previously mentioned animal model of SpA IL-23 could trigger inflammation via IL-17 stimulation but also osteoblast activation through IL-22 activation [27]. Further research is necessary to clarify the pathogenesis of axSpA and the characteristic interaction between inflammation and new bone formation.

Prognostic parameters in axial spondyloarthritis for radiographic progression

In general, AS is a slowly progressing disease. In patients with a mean disease duration of about 20 years, syndesmophytes of the spine were detectable only in about 60% [30]. A growth of syndesmophytes is normally visible on radiographs only over a follow-up period of at least 2 years. However, there is a subgroup of still ill-defined patients who suffer from a more rapid progression. An older retrospective study reported the presence of hip arthritis, elevated erythrocyte sedimentation rate, young age at onset, poor response to nonsteroidal anti-inflammatory drug treatment, and extraspinal manifestations as predictors of a more severe course [31]. The presence of syndesmophytes at baseline seems to be the best predictor for the development of more syndesmophytes [30]. More recently, elevated C-reactive protein was identified as the only relevant parameter predicting progression from nr-axSpA to AS over 2 years [32] and also as a relevant parameter, besides baseline syndesmophytes and smoking, to predict further progression of radiographic damage of the spine [33].

More studies are needed to get a better idea of prognostic factors, which is also crucial for identifying patients who are in need of early, more aggressive therapy.

Genetics of ankylosing spondylitis

Susceptibility to AS has been estimated to be genetically determined in more than 90% of cases, and it has been suggested that, as a result, there might not be a single factor, such as one bacterium, but ubiquitous environmental factors (eg, many different bacteria) [34]. By far the strongest genetic association is with HLA-B27, and more than 100 HLA-B27 subtypes have been described to date. Some of them, such as HLA-B*2706 and HLA-B*2709, do not seem to be associated with the disease, suggesting that minor molecular differences between the molecules might be the key to a better understanding of the pathogenesis. Although differentiation of HLA-B27 subtypes is of research interest, it has no clinical value and should therefore not be applied in daily clinical practice.

Most recently two new genetic loci have been shown to be associated with AS: IL-23 receptor (IL-23R), which is involved in the T-helper cell 17 (Th-17) pathway of chronic immune responses, and endoplasmic reticulum aminopeptidase-1 (ERAP-1), an enzyme that is relevant for the processing of peptides in the cytoplasm [35]. Quite interestingly, an ERAP-1 association has only be found in HLA-B27-positive patients with AS [36], suggesting that ERAP-1 and HLA-B27 might be linked via peptide presentation. The relative contribution of these genes to the susceptibility to AS can be compared by using the population-attributable risk fraction statistic, which is 30–50% for HLA-B27, 26% for ERAP-1, and 9% for IL-23 [35]. Other factors, such as HLA-B60, IL-1A and cytochrome P450 2D6 (*CYP2D6*), have been described as affecting the risk of developing AS, although this is not completely clear.

On the other hand, only about 5% of HLA-B27-positive individuals develop AS. The average risk of developing AS in a first-degree relative (children or sibling) of a patient with AS is about 8%, although only 1% or less of second- and third-degree relatives are affected. The risk can be better estimated when the HLA-B27 status is known: about 12% in HLA-B27-positive first-degree relatives, but less than 1% in HLA-B27-negative relatives (Figure 2.9) [37].

Risk of developing ankylosing spondylitis in a first-degree relative	
HLA-B27 status	**Risk (%)**
Negative	<1
Positive	12
Unknown	8

Figure 2.9 Risk of developing ankylosing spondylitis in a first-degree relative. HLA, human leukocyte antigen. Adapted from Brown et al [37].

References

1 Rudwaleit M, Khan MA, Sieper J. The challenge of diagnosis and classification in early ankylosing spondylitis: do we need new criteria? *Arthritis Rheum.* 2005;52:1000-1008.
2 Dougados M, van der Linden S, Juhlin R, et al. The European Spondylarthropathy Study Group preliminary criteria for the classification of spondylarthropathy. *Arthritis Rheum.* 1991;34:1218-1227.
3 Amor B, Dougados M, Mijiyawa M. [Criteria of the classification of spondylarthropathies]. *Rev Rhum Mal Osteoartic.*1990;57:85-89.
4 Rudwaleit M, van der Heijde D, Landewé R, et al. The development of Assessment of SpondyloArthritis international Society classification criteria for axial spondyloarthritis (part II): validation and final selection. *Ann Rheum Dis.* 2009;68:777-783.
5 Feldtkeller E, Bruckel J, Khan MA. Scientific contributions of ankylosing spondylitis patient advocacy groups. *Curr Opin Rheumatol.* 2000;12:239-247.
6 Rudwaleit M, Haibel H, Baraliakos X, et al. The early disease stage in axial spondylarthritis: results from the German Spondyloarthritis Inception Cohort. *Arthritis Rheum.* 2009;60:717-727.
7 Calin A, Fries JF. Striking prevalence of ankylosing spondylitis in "healthy" w27 positive males and females. *N Engl J Med.* 1975;293:835-839.

8 van der Linden SM, Valkenburg HA, de Jongh BM, Cats A. The risk of developing ankylosing spondylitis in HLA-B27 positive individuals. A comparison of relatives of spondylitis patients with the general population. *Arthritis Rheum.* 1984;27:241-249.

9 Braun J, Listing J, Sieper J, et al. Reply. *Arthritis Rheum.* 2005;52:4049-4059.

10 Gran JT, Husby G, Hordvik M. Prevalence of ankylosing spondylitis in males and females in a young middle-aged population of Tromsø, northern Norway. *Ann Rheum Dis.* 1985;44:359-367.

11 Gofton JP, Robinson HS, Trueman GE. Ankylosing spondylitis in a Canadian Indian population. *Ann Rheum Dis.* 1966;25:525-527.

12 Saraux A, Guillemin F, Guggenbuhl P, et al. Prevalence of spondyloarthropathies in France: 2001. *Ann Rheum Dis.* 2005;64:1431-1435.

13 Guillemin F, Saraux A, Guggenbuhl P, et al. Prevalence of rheumatoid arthritis in France: 2001. *Ann Rheum Dis.* 2005;64:1427-1430.

14 Adomaviciute D, Pileckyte M, Baranauskaite A, Morvan J, Dadoniene J, Guillemin F. Prevalence survey of rheumatoid arthritis and spondyloarthropathy in Lithuania. *Scand J Rheumatol.* 2008;37:113-119.

15 Helmick CG, Felson DT, Lawrence RC, et al; National Arthritis Data Workgroup. Estimates of the prevalence of arthritis and other rheumatic conditions in the United States. Part I. *Arthritis Rheum.* 2008;58:15-25.

16 Sieper J, Rudwaleit M, Khan MA, Braun J. Concepts and epidemiology of spondyloarthritis. *Best Pract Res Clin Rheumatol.* 2006;20:401-417.

17 Reveille JD, Witter JP, Weisman MH. Prevalence of axial spondylarthritis in the United States: Estimates from a cross-sectional survey. *Arthritis Rheum.* 2012;64:905-910.

18 Rudwaleit M, Sieper J. Referral strategies for early diagnosis of axial spondyloarthritis. *Nat Rev Rheumatol.* 2012;8:262-268.

19 Poddubnyy D, Brandt H, Vahldiek J, et al. The frequency of non-radiographic axial spondyloarthritis in relation to symptom duration in patients referred because of chronic back pain: results from the Berlin early spondyloarthritis clinic. *Ann Rheum Dis.* 2012;71:1998-2001.

20 Brewerton DA, Hart FD, Nicholls A, Caffrey M, James DC, Sturrock RD. Ankylosing spondylitis and HL-A 27. *Lancet.* 1973;1:904-907.

21 Sieper J, Braun J, Kingsley GH. Report on the Fourth International Workshop on Reactive Arthritis. *Arthritis Rheum.* 2000;43:720-734.

22 Maksymowych WP. Ankylosing spondylitis--at the interface of bone and cartilage. *J Rheumatol.* 2000;27:2295-2301.

23 Appel H, Kuhne M, Spiekermann S,et al. Immunohistochemical analysis of hip arthritis in ankylosing spondylitis: evaluation of the bone-cartilage interface and subchondral bone marrow. *Arthritis Rheum.* 2006;54:1805-1813.

24 Appel H, Sieper J. Spondyloarthritis at the crossroads of imaging, pathology, and structural damage in the era of biologics. *Curr Rheumatol Rep.* 2008;10:356-363.

25 Appel H, Maier R, Wu P, et al. Analysis of IL-17+ cells in facet joints of patients with spondyloarthritis suggests that the innate immune pathway might be of greater relevance than the Th17-mediated adaptive immune response. *Arthritis Res Ther.* 2011;13:R95.

26 Appel H, Maier R, Bleil J, et al. In situ analysis of interleukin–23– and interleukin–12–positive cells in the spine of patients with ankylosing spondylitis. *Arthritis Rheum.* 2013;65:1522-1529.

27 Sherlock JP, Joyce-Shaikh B, Turner SP, et al. IL-23 induces spondyloarthropathy by acting on ROR-γt+ CD3+CD4-CD8- entheseal resident T cells. *Nat Med.* 2012;18:1069-1076.

28 Sieper J, Appel H, Braun J, Rudwaleit M. Critical appraisal of assessment of structural damage in ankylosing spondylitis: implications for treatment outcomes. *Arthritis Rheum.* 2008;58:649-656.

29 Maksymowych WP, Chiowchanwisawakit P, Clare T, Pedersen SJ, Østergaard M, Lambert RG. Inflammatory lesions of the spine on magnetic resonance imaging predict the development of new syndesmophytes in ankylosing spondylitis: evidence of a relationship between inflammation and new bone formation. *Arthritis Rheum.* 2009;60:93-102.

30 Baraliakos X, Listing J, Rudwaleit M, et al. Progression of radiographic damage in patients with ankylosing spondylitis: defining the central role of syndesmophytes. *Ann Rheum Dis.* 2007;66:910-915.

31 Amor B, Santos RS, Nahal R, Listrat V, Dougados M. Predictive factors for the longterm outcome of spondyloarthropathies. *J Rheumatol.* 1994;21:1883-1887.

32 Poddubnyy D, Rudwaleit M, Haibel H, et al. Rates and predictors of radiographic sacroiliitis progression over 2 years in patients with axial spondyloarthritis. *Ann Rheum Dis.* 2011;70:1369-1374.

33 Poddubnyy D, Haibel H, Listing J, et al. Baseline radiographic damage, elevated acute-phase reactant levels, and cigarette smoking status predict spinal radiographic progression in early axial spondylarthritis. *Arthritis Rheum.* 2012;64:1388-1398.

34 Brown MA, Kennedy LG, MacGregor AJ, et al. Susceptibility to ankylosing spondylitis in twins: the role of genes, HLA, and the environment. *Arthritis Rheum.* 1997;40:1823-1828.

35 Burton PR, Clayton DG, Cardon LR, et al; Wellcome Trust Case Control Consortium; Australo-Anglo-American Spondylitis Consortium (TASC). Association scan of 14,500 nonsynonymous SNPs in four diseases identifies autoimmunity variants. *Nat Genet.* 2007;39:1329-1337.

36 Evans DM, Spencer CC, Pointon JJ, et al; Australo-Anglo-American Spondyloarthritis Consortium (TASC); Wellcome Trust Case Control Consortium 2 (WTCCC2). Interaction between ERAP1 and HLA-B27 in ankylosing spondylitis implicates peptide handling in the mechanism for HLA-B27 in disease susceptibility. *Nat Genet.* 2011;43:761-767.

37 Brown MA, Laval SH, Brophy S, Calin A. Recurrence risk modelling of the genetic susceptibility to ankylosing spondylitis. *Ann Rheum Dis.* 2000;59:883-886.

Chapter 3

Clinical manifestations of axial spondyloarthritis

Inflammatory back pain

The main clinical symptoms in ankylosing spondylitis (AS) are pain and stiffness of the back, predominantly of the lower back and the pelvis, but any part of the spine can be involved. Typical for AS/spondyloarthritis (SpA) is inflammatory back pain (IBP), which is defined clinically and not by laboratory tests, such as C-reactive protein (CRP) or erythrocyte sedimentation rate (ESR). Patients complain about morning stiffness of the back, with improvement on exercise but not by rest. In addition, or alternatively, they report awakening at night, mostly in the second half of the night, because of back pain, which improves on getting up and moving around (Figure 3.1). Furthermore, back pain should be chronic (>3 months duration) not acute, and it should occur for the first time before the age of 45 years because the disease starts at a young age; this also helps to differentiate it from degenerative spine disease, the prevalence of which increases with age. Most patients report a mixture of pain and stiffness in the spine, although either can be the main or only symptom.

Characteristics of inflammatory back pain
Morning stiffness of the back >30 min
Awakening in the second half of the night because of back pain
Improvement of pain and stiffness by exercise but not by rest
Chronic back pain (>3 months duration) starting at an age <45 years

Figure 3.1 Characteristics of inflammatory back pain.

J. Sieper and J. Braun, *Clinician's Manual on Axial Spondyloarthritis*,
DOI: 10.1007/978-1-907673-85-6_3, © Springer Healthcare 2014

Various sets of criteria for IBP have been proposed and applied combining the parameters mentioned above and shown in Figure 3.2 [1–3]. They also performed well when investigated in studies, although all have a limited sensitivity and specificity. A sensitivity of no more than 80% implies that 20% of patients with AS do not complain about characteristic IBP, and a specificity no higher than 80% means that 20% of control patients (eg, patients with mechanically induced low back pain) complain about, for example, morning stiffness with improvement through exercise [4]. Nevertheless, IBP is an important clinical criterion in AS/SpA.

Restriction of spinal mobility

Further in the course of the disease, syndesmophytes and ossification of the facet joints can develop, resulting in restriction of spinal mobility. The long-term outcome is strongly determined by restriction of spinal mobility. However, not all patients with AS have syndesmophytes. In patients with AS with a disease (symptom) duration of less than 10 years syndesmophytes are detectable in only about 25%, and in patients with a mean disease duration of more than 20 years syndesmophytes are visible on radiographs in about 60% [5,6]. A recent study showed that both disease activity and radiographic damage of the spine determine function independently, with disease activity being more relevant earlier in the course of the disease [7]. Measurement and documentation of

Inflammatory back pain defined according to various criteria		
Calin et al [1]	**Rudwaleit et al [2]**	**IBP experts (ASAS) [3]**
age at onset <40 yrs	morning stiffness >30 min	age at onset <40 yrs
duration of back pain >3 months	improvement with exercise, not with rest	insidious onset
		improvement with exercise
insidious onset	awakening at 2nd half of the night because of pain	no improvement with rest
morning stiffness		pain at night (with improvement upon getting up)
improvement with exercise	alternating buttock pain	
IBP if 4 / 5 are present	**IBP if 2 / 4 are present**	**IBP if 4 / 5 are present**

Figure 3.2 Inflammatory back pain defined according to various criteria. ASAS, Assessment in SpondyloArthritis international Society; IBP, inflammatory back pain. Adapted from Calin et al [1], Rudwaleit et al [2], Sieper et al [3].

spinal mobility, as shown in Figures 3.3–3.7, are recommended in the follow-up of patients with AS.

Modified Schober test to assess motion of the lumbar spine

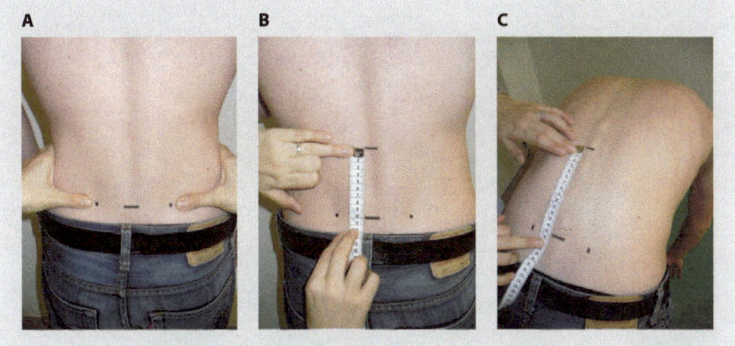

Figure 3.3 Modified Schober test to assess motion of the lumbar spine. A, the patient stands erect and the clinician marks an imaginary line connecting both posterior superior iliac spines (close to the dimples of Venus); **B,** another mark is placed 10 cm above; **C,** the patient bends forward maximally, and the difference is measured. The best of two attempts is recorded and the increase in centimeters is recorded to the nearest 0.1 cm.

Measuring lateral spinal flexion

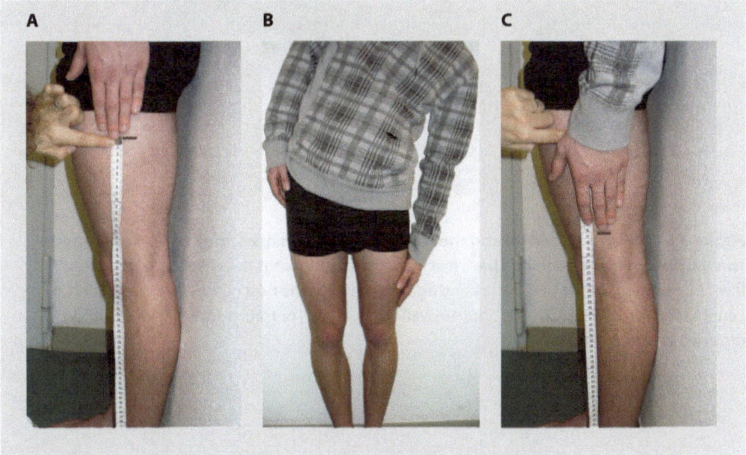

Figure 3.4 Measuring lateral spinal flexion. A, the patient rests their heels and back against the wall, with no flexion in the knees and without bending forward and the clinician marks the thigh; **B,** the patient bends sideways without bending their knees or lifting their heels; **C,** the clinician places a second mark and records the difference.

Measuring cervical and thoracic spine extension: occiput-to-wall and tragus-to-wall distance

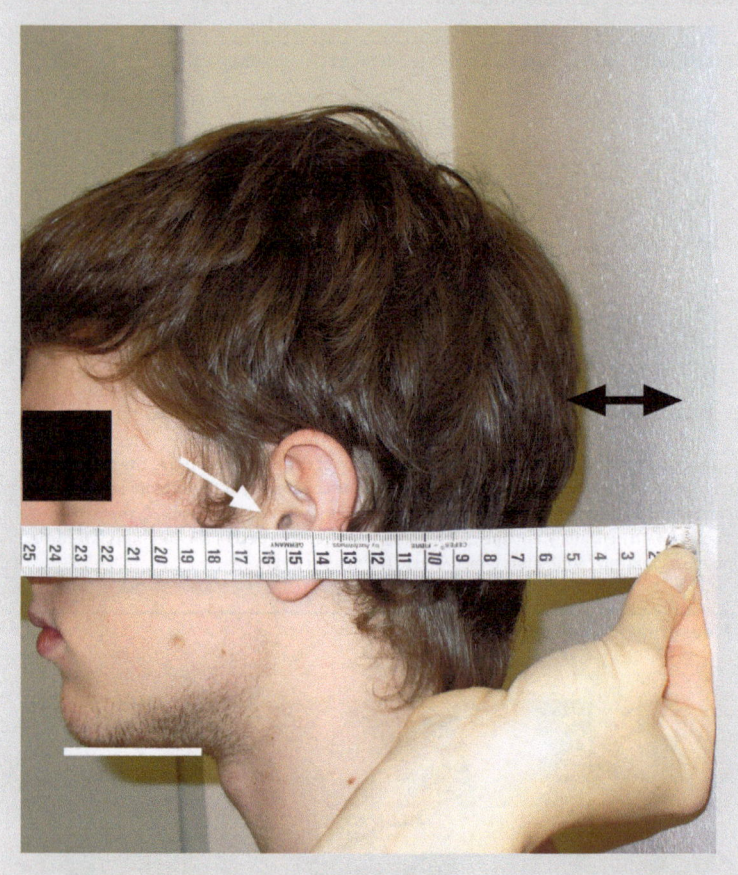

Figure 3.5 Measuring cervical and thoracic spine extension: occiput-to-wall and tragus-to-wall distance. The heels and back rest against the wall, with the chin at usual carrying level. The patient tries to touch the head against the wall. The best of two tries is recorded in centimeters (eg, 10.2 cm). The occiput-to-wall (black arrow) or tragus-to-wall (white arrow) distance can be measured.

Measuring cervical rotation to assess neck mobility in patients with ankylosing spondylitis

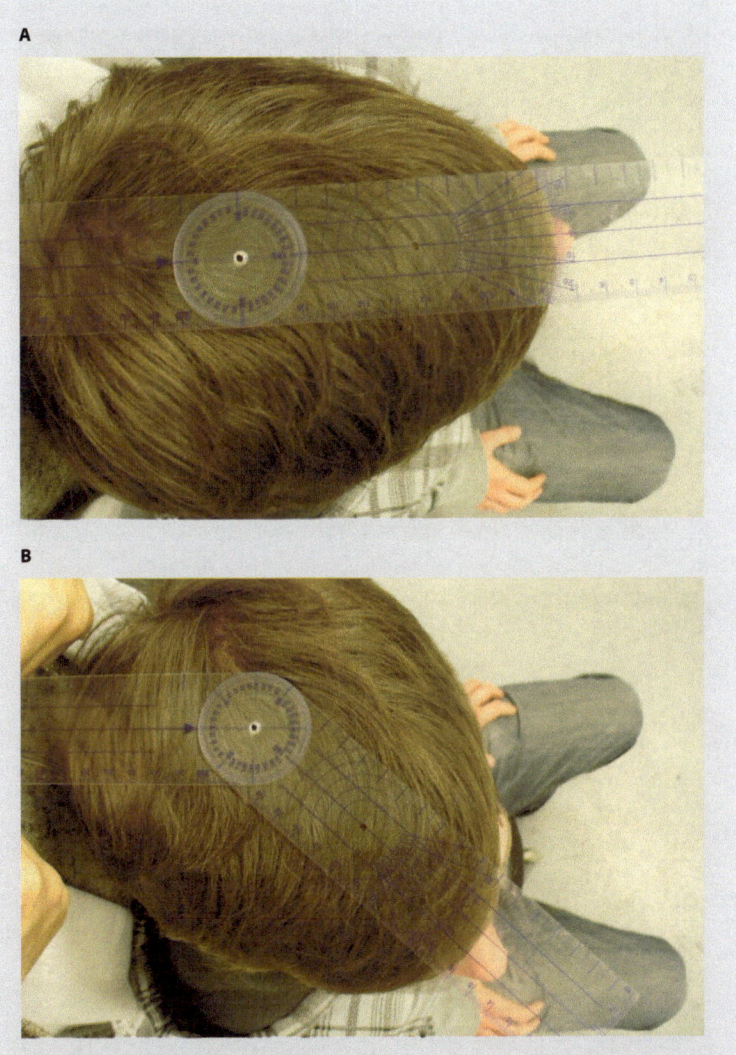

Figure 3.6 Measuring cervical rotation to assess neck mobility in patients with ankylosing spondylitis. A, the patient sits straight on a chair, chin level, hands on the knees. The assessor places a goniometer at the top of the head in line with the nose; **B,** the assessor asks the patient to rotate the neck maximally to the left, follows with the goniometer, and records the angle between the sagittal plane and the new plane after rotation. A second reading is taken and the best of the two is recorded for the left side. The procedure is repeated for the right side. The mean of left and right is recorded in degrees (0–90°) (normal >70°).

Chest expansion

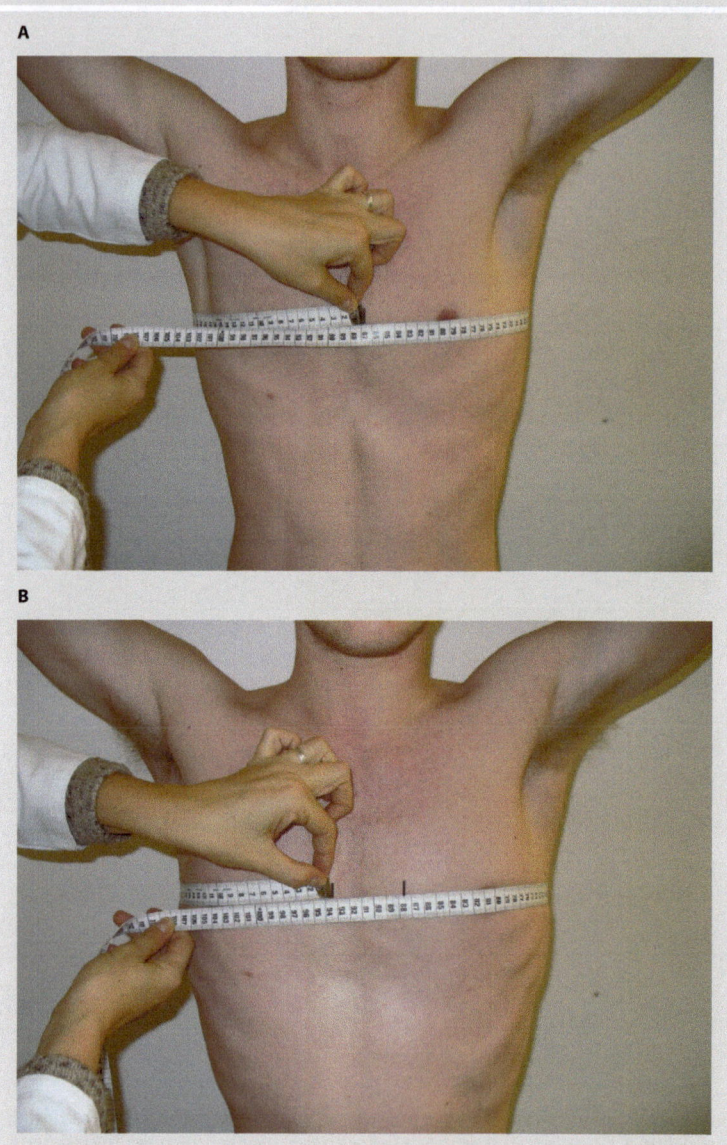

Figure 3.7 Chest expansion. The patient rests his/her hands on or behind the head. The chest is measured at the fourth intercostal level anteriorly. **A,** the maximal inspiration is recorded; **B,** the maximal expiration is recorded. The difference is recorded in centimeters (eg, 4.3 cm) and the best of two tries is noted.

In addition to restriction of spinal mobility, patients can develop flexion contractures of hip and knee joints, which together result in a characteristic posture for advanced disease in patients with AS (see Figure 1.1A).

Extraspinal rheumatic manifestations

Peripheral arthritis

Peripheral arthritis occurs frequently, but often transiently, in axial spondyloarthritis (axSpA) and presents typically as an asymmetrical arthritis and/or as an arthritis predominantly of the lower limbs (Figure 3.8). In a cohort of patients with AS with a mean symptom duration of 18 years, 58% of patients reported a peripheral arthritis [8]. This figure was slightly lower in an AS cohort with a symptom duration of less than 10 years, with 37.4% of patients reporting arthritis, but only 14.4% of patients reporting it at the time of presentation [5]. The pattern of peripheral joint involvement in one study was oligoarthritis (fewer than five joints) in 55%, monoarthritis in 24%, and polyarthritis in 21% [8].

Enthesitis

Enthesitis (inflammation at the insertion of tendons, ligaments, or capsules into bone) is also a frequent manifestation in AS and nonradiological axial spondyloarthritis (nr-axSpA) and occurred in 50% of a cohort with long-standing AS and in 39.4% of a cohort with shorter disease duration [5,8]. The percentage of patients with enthesitis at presentation was 21% in the latter cohort. The lower limbs are most frequently affected, especially at the insertion of Achilles' tendon and/or the plantar fascia at the calcaneus (Figure 3.9); however, inflammation is possible at any enthesial site.

Enthesitis in peripheral joints

The sites affected by inflammation in peripheral joints can be both the synovium and the insertion of tendons/ligaments at bone. Figure 3.10 shows a good example of both subchondral bone marrow edema and effusion in a patient with SpA with gonarthritis, compared with a patient with rheumatoid arthritis with no bone marrow edema [9]. This implies that

Acute gonarthritis in a patient with peripheral spondyloarthritis

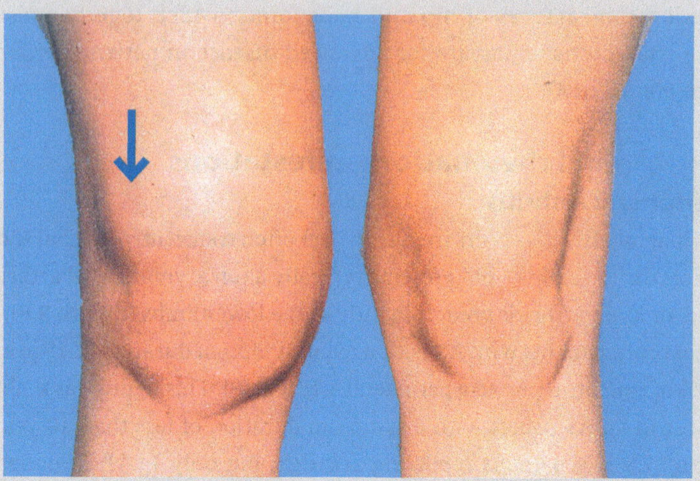

Figure 3.8 Acute gonarthritis in a patient with peripheral spondyloarthritis. The knee on the left shows a patient with peripheral spondyloarthritis (arrow) while the knee on the right is normal. Reproduced with permission from © ASAS [www.asas-group.org]. All Rights Reserved.

a peripheral joint in SpA might not be swollen, only painful (especially pain on local pressure and, if accessible, on movement).

Hip and shoulder joints

Involvement of the hip and shoulder joints is frequent, but often regarded as part of the axial skeleton manifestation and not as peripheral arthritis. Hip involvement was reported in 27% of patients with AS with longstanding disease [8] and it can be expected that about 5% of patients with AS have to undergo hip joint replacement in the course of their disease as a result of arthritis of the hip and secondary osteoarthritis. In one study, shoulder pain was reported in 3.5% and shoulder involvement by clinical evaluation in 25% [10]. Rotator cuff tendonitis and enthesitis at the insertion of the supraspinatus tendon at the greater tuberosity of the humerus (Figure 3.11) and enthesitis at the acromial origin of the deltoid muscle were the most frequently found abnormalities, when patients were examined by magnetic resonance imaging (MRI) [10]. Bone marrow edema was the most characteristic finding while effusion was rare.

Enthesitis in the right heel of a patient

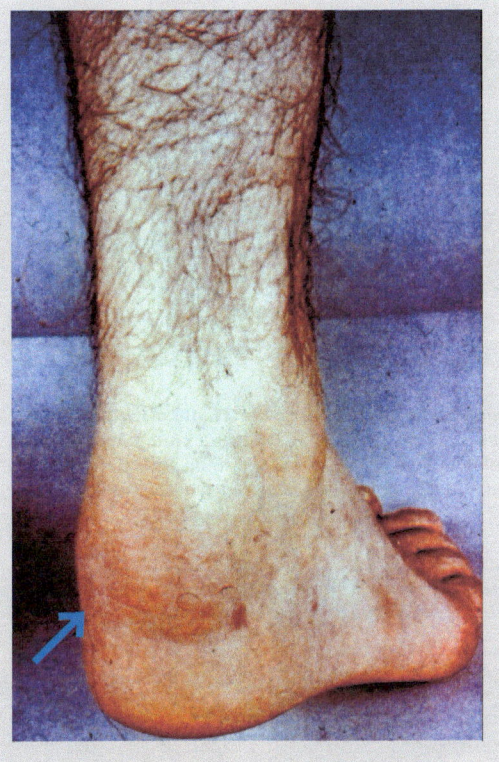

Figure 3.9 Enthesitis in the right heel of a patient. Insertion of Achilles' tendon at calcaneus.

Dactylitis

Dactylitis is a swelling of a finger or toe as a consequence of a tendovaginitis (Figure 3.12). It is typical for the whole group of SpA but it is more rare in AS (dactylitis in 6.3% in one study [8]) than it is in psoriatic arthritis.

Extraarticular locations

Uveitis anterior is the most frequent extraarticular location in AS, which occurs in about 30% of patients with AS. This percentage was lower (21%) in patients with AS with a symptom duration of less than 10 years. The percentage of patients with uveitis at presentation is rather small (1.7% in

Spondyloarthritis and rheumatoid arthritis of the knee by MRI

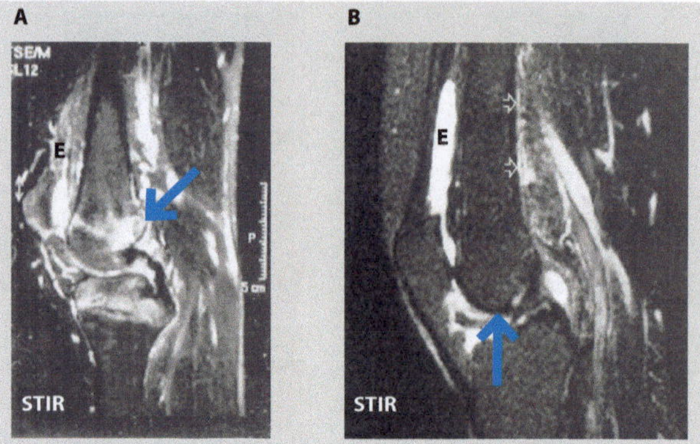

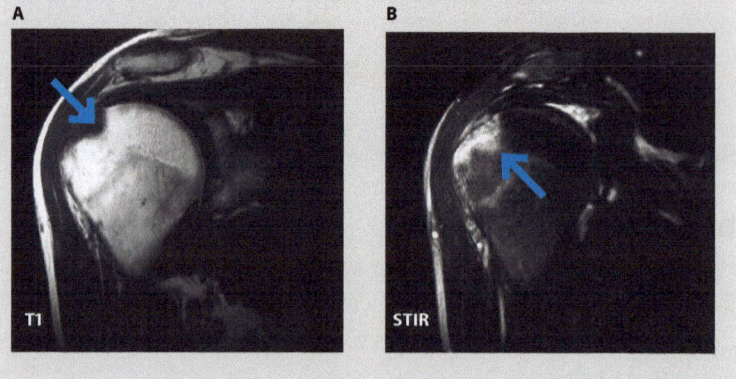

Figure 3.10 Spondyloarthritis and rheumatoid arthritis of the knee by MRI.
A, spondyloarthritis with osteitis (arrow) and effusion (E); **B,** rheumatoid arthritis with synovitis (arrow) and effusion (E). STIR, short tau inversion recovery. Reproduced with permission from © John Wiley and Sons 2013, McGonagle et al [9]. All Rights Reserved.

Supraspinatus enthesitis at the humerus head in a patient with ankylosing spondylitis as seen by MRI

Figure 3.11 Supraspinatus enthesitis at the humerus head in a patient with ankylosing spondylitis as seen by MRI. A, bone marrow edema: hypointense on T1; **B,** bone marrow edema: hyperintense on STIR. STIR, short tau inversion recovery. Reproduced with permission from © John Wiley and Sons 2013, Lambert et al [10]. All Rights Reserved.

one study) [5]. The typical clinical picture of uveitis is predominantly anterior, unilateral, sudden in onset, limited in duration, and often alternating from one eye to the other (Figure 3.13) [11].

The presence or history of psoriasis is reported in about 10% of patients with AS and the presence or history of inflammatory bowel disease is reported in 3–10%, with an increasing frequency found over time.

Dactylitis in a patient with psoriasis

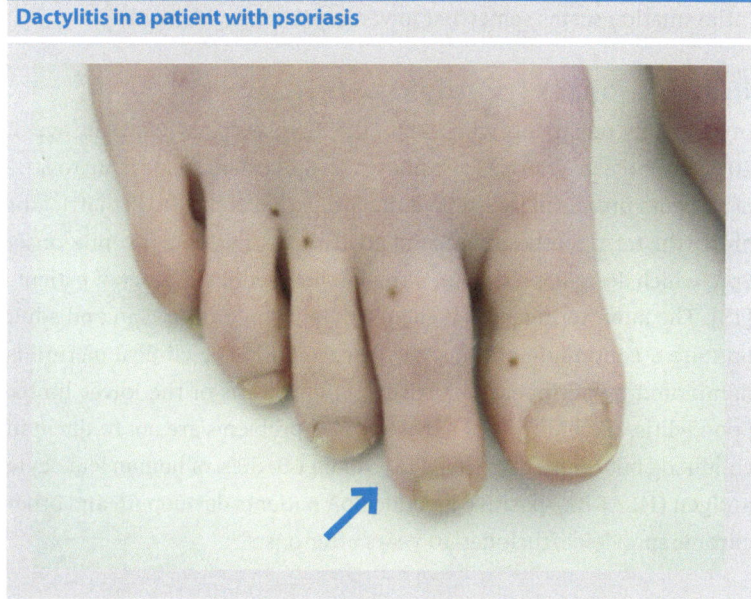

Figure 3.12 Dactylitis in a patient with psoriasis. Swelling of the second toe in a patient with psoriasis.

Clinical characteristics of uveitis anterior in ankylosing spondylitis

Acute (self-limiting)
Unilateral
Sudden in onset (painful and red eye)
Alternating from one eye to the other

Figure 3.13 Clinical characteristics of uveitis anterior in ankylosing spondylitis.

Comparison of clinical manifestations between ankylosing spondylitis and nonradiographic axial spondyloarthritis

When the frequency and intensity of spinal, extraspinal, and extraarticular manifestation were compared they were very similar, underlining that both axSpA stages belong to the same disease [5,12]. However, the male/female ratio is higher in patients with AS and the burden of inflammation seems somewhat lower in patients with nr-axSpA.

Juvenile-onset spondyloarthritis

In up to 20% of patients with axSpA the disease starts before the age of 20 years and a diagnosis of juvenile-onset SpA can be made in up to 50% of patients presenting with juvenile idiopathic arthritis. Pediatricians prefer the term "enthesitis-related arthritis" rather than juvenile-onset SpA, which describes a similar, although not identical, subset of patients [13]. The latter term makes it clearer that juvenile-onset SpA and adult SpA are a continuum of the same disease [14]. The clinical picture is dominated by peripheral arthritis and enthesitis of the lower limbs. Spondylitis, sacroiliitis, and extraarticular problems are not frequent in childhood but evolve over time [15]. About 60–80% of human leukocyte antigen (HLA)-B27-positive juvenile SpA patients develop AS and other chronic spondyloarthritides 10 years after onset.

References

1   Calin A, Porta J, Fries JF, Schurman DJ. Clinical history as a screening test for ankylosing spondylitis. *JAMA*. 1977;237:2613-2614.

2   Rudwaleit M, Metter A, Listing J, Sieper J, Braun J. Inflammatory back pain in ankylosing spondylitis: a reassessment of the clinical history for application as classification and diagnostic criteria. *Arthritis Rheum*. 2006;54:569-578.

3   Sieper J, van der Heijde D, Landewé R, et al. New criteria for inflammatory back pain in patients with chronic back pain: a real patient exercise of the Assessment in SpondyloArthritis international Society (ASAS). *Ann Rheum Dis*. 2009;68:784-788.

4   Rudwaleit M, van der Heijde D, Khan MA, Braun J, Sieper J. How to diagnose axial spondyloarthritis early. *Ann Rheum Dis*. 2004;63:535-543.

5   Rudwaleit M, Haibel H, Baraliakos X, et al. The early disease stage in axial spondyloarthritis: results from the German spondyloarthritis inception cohort. *Arthritis Rheum*. 2009;60:717-727.

6   Baraliakos X, Listing J, Rudwaleit M, et al. Progression of radiographic damage in patients with ankylosing spondylitis: defining the central role of syndesmophytes. *Ann Rheum Dis*. 2007;66:910-915.

7 Landewé R, Dougados M, Mielants H, van der Tempel H, van der Heijde D. Physical function in ankylosing spondylitis is independently determined by both disease activity and radiographic damage of the spine. *Ann Rheum Dis*. 2009;68:863-867.

8 Vander Cruyssen B, Ribbens C, Boonen A, et al. The epidemiology of ankylosing spondylitis and the commencement of anti-TNF therapy in daily rheumatology practice. *Ann Rheum Dis*. 2007;66:1072-1077.

9 McGonagle D, Gibbon W, O'Connor P, Green M, Pease C, Emery P. Characteristic magnetic resonance imaging entheseal changes of knee synovitis in spondylarthropathy. *Arthritis Rheum*. 1998;41:694-700.

10 Lambert RG, Dhillon SS, Jhangri GS, et al. High prevalence of symptomatic enthesiopathy of the shoulder in ankylosing spondylitis: deltoid origin involvement constitutes a hallmark of disease. *Arthritis Rheum*. 2004;51:681-690.

11 Zeboulon N, Dougados M, Gossec L. Prevalence and characteristics of uveitis in the spondyloarthropathies: a systematic literature review. *Ann Rheum Dis*. 2008;67:955-959.

12 Dougados M, d'Agostino MA, Benessiano J, et al. The DESIR cohort: a 10-year follow-up of early inflammatory back pain in France: study design and baseline characteristics of the 708 recruited patients. *Joint Bone Spine*. 2011;78:598-603.

13 Verstappen SM, Jacobs JW, van der Heijde DM, et al. Utility and direct costs: ankylosing spondylitis compared with rheumatoid arthritis. *Ann Rheum Dis*. 2007;66:727-731.

14 Burgos-Vargas R. The assessment of the spondyloarthritis international society concept and criteria for the classification of axial spondyloarthritis and peripheral spondyloarthritis: A critical appraisal for the pediatric rheumatologist. *Pediatric Rheumatology Online J*. 2012;10:14.

15 Burgos-Vargas R, Vázquez-Mellado J. The early clinical recognition of juvenile-onset ankylosing spondylitis and its differentiation from juvenile rheumatoid arthritis. *Arthritis Rheum*. 1995;38:835-844.

Chapter 4

Diagnosis of axial spondyloarthritis

The modified New York criteria

According to the modified New York criteria, which are still widely used, the hallmark for the diagnosis of ankylosing spondylitis (AS) has been the detection of sacroiliitis by radiographs (Figure 4.1) [1,2]. Sacroiliitis is graded using a scoring system as shown in Figure 4.2 [3]. A diagnosis of AS can be made if sacroiliitis grade 2 bilaterally or grade 3 or higher unilaterally is present together with one clinical criterion, such as the presence of the clinical symptom inflammatory back pain or restriction of spinal mobility. As spinal involvement with the development of syndesmophytes normally occurs later in the course of the disease and as the spine is rarely affected without the sacroiliac (SI) joint, radiographic changes of the spine are not part of these diagnostic criteria. Examples of normal and abnormal sacroiliac joints are shown in Figures 4.3–4.5.

Modified New York criteria for ankylosing spondylitis
1. Clinical criteria
Low back pain and stiffness >3 months which improves with exercise, but is not relieved by rest
Limitation of motion of the lumbar spine in both the sagittal and frontal planes
Limitation of chest expansion relative to normal values correlated for age and sex
2. Radiological criterion
Sacroiliitis grade ≥2 bilaterally or grade 3–4 unilaterally
Definite AS if the radiological criterion is associated with at least 1 clinical criterion.

Figure 4.1 Modified New York criteria for ankylosing spondylitis. AS, ankylosing spondylitis. Adapted from van der Linden et al [2].

J. Sieper and J. Braun, *Clinician's Manual on Axial Spondyloarthritis*, DOI: 10.1007/978-1-907673-85-6_4, © Springer Healthcare 2014

Grading of radiographic sacroiliitis

Grade 0	Normal
Grade 1	Suspicious changes
Grade 2	Minimal abnormality – small localized areas with erosion or sclerosis, without alteration in the joint width
Grade 3	Unequivocal abnormality – moderate or advanced sacroiliitis with one or more of: erosions, evidence of sclerosis, widening, narrowing, or partial ankylosis
Grade 4	Severe abnormality – total ankylosis

Figure 4.2 Grading of radiographic sacroiliitis. Adapted from Bennett and Burch [3].

Sacroiliitis grade 0 normal

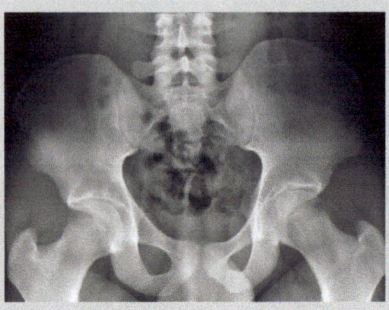

Figure 4.3 Sacroiliitis grade 0 normal. Reproduced with permission from © ASAS [www.asas-group.org]. All Rights Reserved.

Sacroiliitis grade 1 and 2

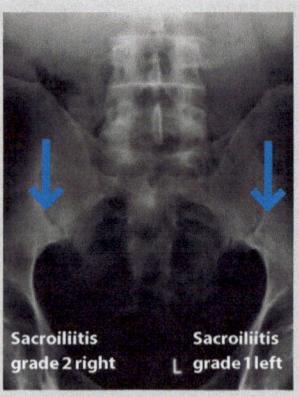

Figure 4.4 Sacroiliitis grade 1 and 2. A patient with grade 1 sacroiliitis on the left and grade 2 sacroiliitis on the right. Reproduced with permission from © ASAS [www.asas-group.org]. All Rights Reserved.

Sacroiliitis grade 3 bilaterally

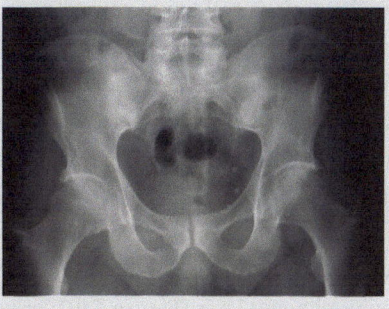

Figure 4.5 Sacroiliitis grade 3 bilaterally. Reproduced with permission from © ASAS [www.asas-group.org]. All Rights Reserved.

Delay between onset of symptoms and diagnosis

There is currently an unacceptably long delay between the first occurrence of AS symptoms and a diagnosis of AS being made 5–10 years afterwards (see Figure 2.4) [4,5]. This results in young patients with chronic back pain frequently consulting many different physicians, having redundant and potentially expensive diagnostic procedures and treatments and, most importantly, having a major delay in starting effective therapy.

There are two major reasons for such a delay: the first is that there is certainly a low awareness of AS among non-rheumatologists and it can also be seen as a major challenge for any physician in primary care to think of and identify patients with inflammatory spine disease among the large group of patients with chronic back pain, most often of other origin. To change this, the awareness of the disease among non-specialists has to be increased and effective programs for screening of patients with chronic back pain for inflammatory spinal disease have to be incorporated into primary care. Possible solutions and first results are presented later in the chapter (see "Screening for axial SpA" on page 40).

Second, radiographic sacroiliitis is usually a requirement for making a diagnosis of AS according to the modified New York criteria, as discussed earlier. However, radiographic changes indicate chronic changes and damage of the bone, and are the consequence of inflammation and not active inflammation itself. AS is a slowly progressive disease in terms of radiographic changes, and definite sacroiliitis on plain radiographs appears relatively late, often following several years of continuous or relapsing inflammation [6]. Figure 4.6 shows an estimated correlation between length of symptoms and the development of radiographic changes [6]. Only a small proportion of patients will already have radiographic sacroiliitis at their first visit to the doctor, probably as a result of ongoing subclinical inflammation (Figure 4.6A). After about 5 years roughly half the patients will already have radiographic sacroiliitis, but the other half will not (Figure 4.6B). A smaller proportion of patients develop radiographic changes later (Figure 4.6C) or never (Figure 4.6D). Thus, for early diagnosis radiographic changes of the SI joints have a very limited role.

Classification and diagnosis of axial spondyloarthritis including nonradiographic axial spondyloarthritis

In early disease with no definite radiographic changes, active inflammation of SI joints can normally be visualized using magnetic resonance

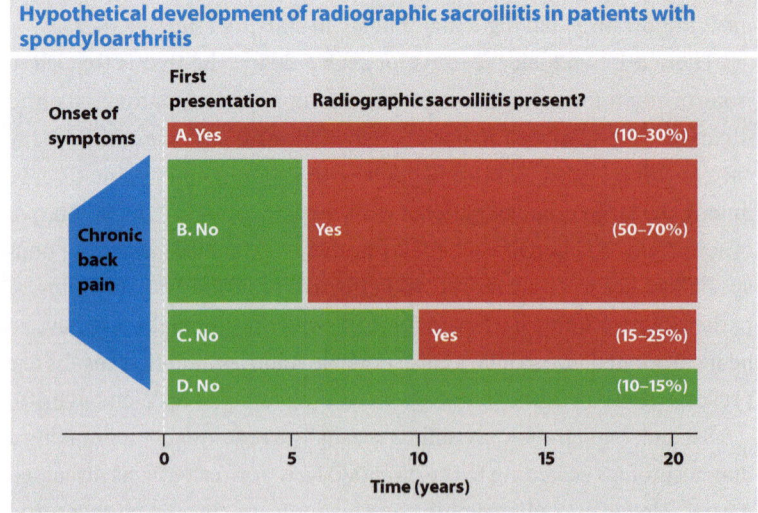

Figure 4.6 Hypothetical development of radiographic sacroiliitis in patients with spondyloarthritis. Reproduced with permission from © John Wiley and Sons 2013, Rudwaleit et al [6]. All Rights Reserved.

imaging (MRI) technology. The hallmark of a "positive MRI" is the presence of subchondral bone marrow edema, as shown in Figure 4.7 and discussed in more detail in Chapter 5 [7,8]. Clinical experience but also limited data suggest that a good proportion of patients with inflammation of the SI joints on MRI, but normal or suspicious radiographs, will develop radiographic sacroiliitis later on, which therefore evolves to AS [9]. Thus, Assessment in SpondyloArthritis international Society (ASAS) has proposed that all patients with spondyloarthritis (SpA) with predominant axial involvement, irrespective of the presence or absence of radiographic changes, should be considered as belonging to one disease continuum (Figure 4.8) [6]. Furthermore, the term "nonradiographic axial SpA" should be used for the group of patients with early axial SpA (axSpA) without radiographic evidence of a sacroiliitis. Such a term is also preferable compared with "undifferentiated (ax)SpA" because this subgroup is now well defined and can be diagnosed with no problems.

Following this reasoning, new criteria for the classification of axSpA have been developed and are shown in Figures 4.9 and 4.10 [10]. Sacroiliitis, as seen on imaging, is still a crucial part of these criteria, but it can be detected by either radiographs (indicating chronic damage) or MRI (which is new!), showing active inflammation of the SI joint. Thus, radiographic sacroiliitis, as defined by the modified New York criteria, is part of, but not essential to, the classification. In addition to identifying

Acute sacroiliitis

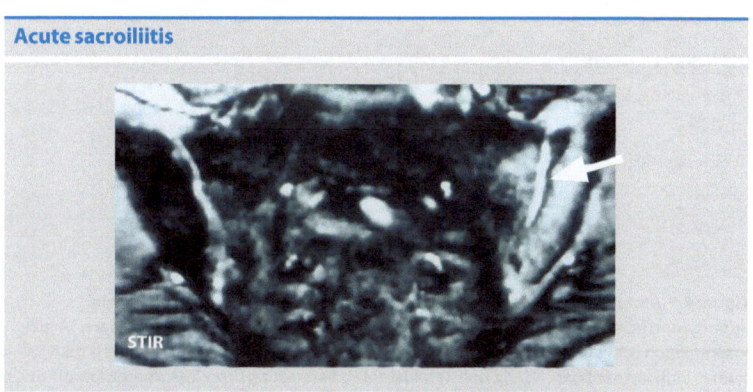

Figure 4.7 Acute sacroiliitis. Patient with acute sacroiliitis (arrow). Reproduced with permission from © John Wiley and Sons 2013, Braun et al [8]. All Rights Reserved.

sacroiliitis by imaging, one of the typical features of SpA has to be present (Figure 4.9). Restriction of spinal mobility, which is one of the clinical criteria for the modified New York criteria, is no longer part of the new criteria. Patients can also be classified as axSpA in the absence of imaging results if three clinical parameters, including human leukocyte antigen (HLA)-B27 positivity, are present.

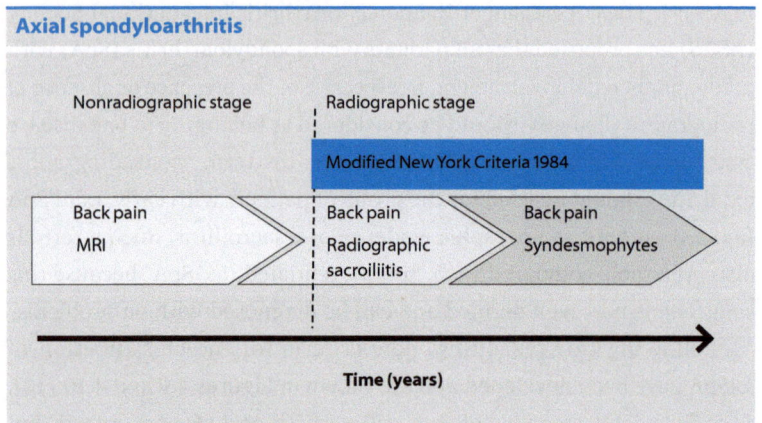

Axial spondyloarthritis

Nonradiographic stage | Radiographic stage

Modified New York Criteria 1984

Back pain
MRI

Back pain
Radiographic
sacroiliitis

Back pain
Syndesmophytes

Time (years)

Figure 4.8 Axial spondyloarthritis. Reproduced with permission from © John Wiley and Sons 2013, Rudwaleit et al [6]. All Rights Reserved.

Assessment in SpondyloArthritis international Society criteria for axial spondyloarthritis in patients with back pain ≥3 months and age at onset <45 years

Sacroiliitis by MRI* or radiographs† plus one SpA clinical criterion	or	**HLA-B27** plus two SpA clinical criteria
SpA clinical criteria		
Inflammatory back pain		Psoriasis
Arthritis		Inflammatory bowel disease
Enthesitis (heel)		Good response to NSAIDs
Uveitis		Family history of spondyloarthritis
Dactylitis		Positive HLA-B27
		Positive C-reactive protein

Figure 4.9 Assessment in SpondyloArthritis international Society criteria for axial spondyloarthritis in patients with back pain ≥3 months and age at onset <45 years. *Active inflammation compatible with sacroiliitis; †According to the modified New York criteria. HLA, human leukocyte antigen; NSAID, nonsteroidal anti-inflammatory drug; SpA, spondyloarthritis. Reproduced with permission from © BMJ Publishing Group Ltd. 2013, Rudwaleit et al [10]. All Rights Reserved.

Variables used in the Assessment in SpondyloArthritis international Society criteria for classification of axial spondyloarthritis

Clinical criterion	Definition
Inflammatory back pain	According to experts: four out of five of the following parameters present:
	1. age at onset <40 years
	2. insidious onset
	3. improvement with exercise
	4. no improvement with rest
	5. pain at night (with improvement upon getting up)
Arthritis	Past or present active synovitis diagnosed by a doctor
Family history	Presence in first-degree or second-degree relatives of any of the following:
	a. ankylosing spondylitis
	b. psoriasis
	c. uveitis
	d. reactive arthritis
	e. inflammatory bowel disease
Psoriasis	Past or present psoriasis diagnosed by a doctor
Inflammatory bowel disease	Past or present Crohn's disease or ulcerative colitis diagnosed by a doctor
Dactylitis	Past or present dactylitis diagnosed by a doctor
Enthesitis	Heel enthesitis: past or present spontaneous pain or tenderness at examination of the site of the insertion of Achilles' tendon or plantar fascia at the calcaneus
Uveitis anterior	Past or present uveitis anterior, confirmed by an ophthalmologist
Good response to NSAIDs	24–48 hours after a full dose of a NSAID the back pain is not present anymore or much better
HLA-B27	Positive testing according to standard laboratory techniques
Elevated CRP	CRP above upper normal limit, in the presence of back pain, after exclusion of other causes for elevated CRP concentration
Sacroiliitis by radiographs	Bilateral grade 2–4 or unilateral grade 3–4, according to the modified New York criteria
Sacroiliitis by MRI	Active inflammatory lesions of sacroiliac joints with definite bone marrow edema/ostitis suggestive of sacroiliitis associated with spondyloarthritis

Figure 4.10 Variables used in the Assessment in SpondyloArthritis international Society criteria for classification of axial spondyloarthritis. CRP, C-reactive protein; HLA, human leukocyte antigen; NSAID, nonsteroidal anti-inflammatory drug. Reproduced with permission from © BMJ Publishing Group Ltd. 2013, Rudwaleit et al [10]. All Rights Reserved.

Classification criteria are developed to get a clear "yes" or "no" answer from a given patient, normally to decide on whether the patient would be suitable for a clinical study as patient populations need to be homogeneous for studies. In daily clinical practice such a clear decision is often not possible (and not always wanted), especially early in the course of the disease, and a more flexible approach is necessary. Figure 4.11 shows the diagnostic algorithm for axSpA proposed by ASAS [11,12]. As the sensitivity and specificity for each of the parameters shown in this algorithm are known (Figure 4.12), the posttest probability for the diagnosis can be calculated if one or several of these parameters are positive [11]. For this the pretest probability that a patient with chronic back pain seen in primary care has axSpA has to be known before any further details about clinical, laboratory, or imaging parameters are available. As a result of the relatively low pretest probability of about 5% (ie, 1 in 20 chronic back pain patients has axSpA) [13], under these circumstances a combination of several clinical (such as inflammatory back pain, enthesitis, uveitis, and peripheral arthritis), laboratory (such as HLA-B27 or C-reactive protein [CRP]) and imaging parameters (radiographs or MRI) are necessary for an early diagnosis.

The more advanced the disease and the more chronic damage that has already occurred (such as syndesmophytes), the easier it is for a diagnosis to be made in the presence of just a few parameters (such as positive radiographs), but not early in the course of the disease. Of note, inflammatory back pain is not used as an essential entry criterion in the diagnostic algorithm shown in Figure 4.11 because the sensitivity for this symptom is not higher than 80%, so 20% of the patients with the disease would be missed if inflammatory back pain were regarded as essential.

Subsequently we proposed a slightly modified and even more flexible diagnostic approach [11]. If the sensitivity and specificity of a single parameter for a given disease (in this case axSpA) are known, the likelihood ratio (LR) can be easily calculated (Figure 4.12), which is a good indicator for the diagnostic value of a parameter: the higher the LR, the higher the value of this parameter for diagnosis. If several parameters are present the LRs can be multiplied and the posttest probability calculated. Figures 4.13 and 4.14 give two examples of a combination

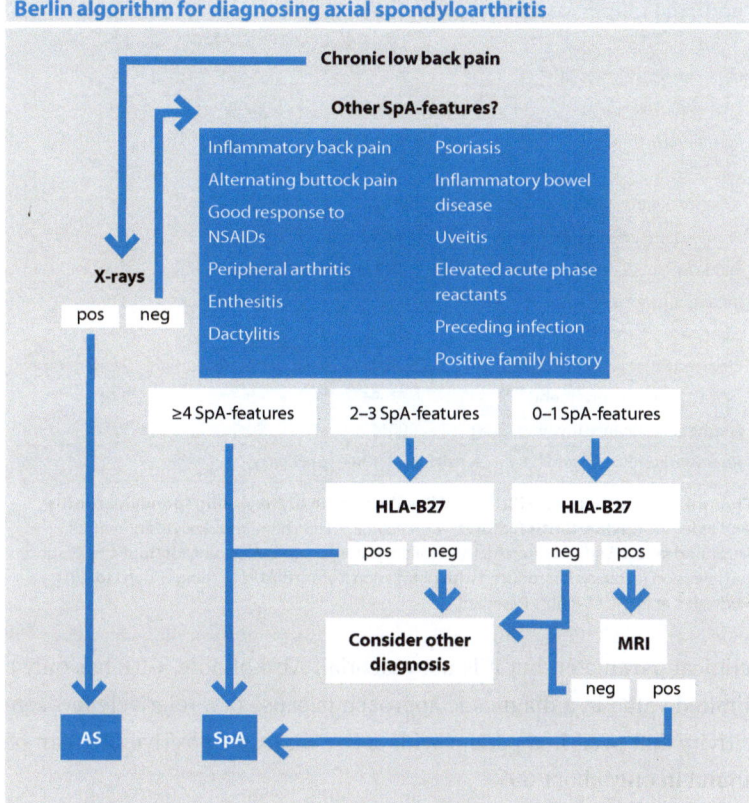

Figure 4.11 Assessment in SpondyloArthritis international Society modification of the Berlin algorithm for diagnosing axial spondyloarthritis. AS, ankylosing spondylitis; HLA, human leukocyte antigen; neg, negative; NSAID, nonsteroidal anti-inflammatory drugs; pos, positive; SpA, spondyloarthritis. Reproduced with permission from © BMJ Publishing Group Ltd. 2013, Rudwaleit et al [11], van den Berg et al [12]. All Rights Reserved.

of different SpA-typical parameters and the resulting posttest probability that a diagnosis of axSpA is present, in the absence of radiographic sacroiliitis [6]. As can be seen from the LR values (Figures 4.12–4.14) a positive MRI and a positive HLA-B27 are the best single parameters in this diagnostic pyramid. The relevance of these two parameters, especially for early diagnosis, is also reflected in the ASAS classification criteria (see Figure 4.9) [10]. Using this approach in patients with chronic back pain, the clinical symptom of inflammatory back pain is one (important)

Sensitivity, specificity, and likelihood ratio of ankylosing spondyloarthritis and axial spondyloarthritis features

	Sensitivity (%)	Specificity (%)	LR+
Inflammatory back pain	71–75	75–80	3.7
Enthesitis (heel pain)	16–37	89–94	3.4
Peripheral arthritis	40–62	90–98	4.0
Dactylitis	12–24	96–98	4.5
Anterior uveitis	10–22	97–99	7.3
Positive family history for SpA	7–36	93–99	6.4
Psoriasis	10–20	95–97	4.0
Inflammatory bowel disease	5–8	97–99	4.0
Good response to NSAIDs	61–77	80–85	5.1
Elevated acute phase reactants	38–69	67–80	2.5
HLA-B27 (axial involvement)	83–96	90–96	9.0
Magnetic resonance imaging (STIR)	90*	90*	9.0
Positive likelihood ratio (LR+) = sensitivity / (100 – specificity)			

Figure 4.12 Sensitivity, specificity, and likelihood ratio of ankylosing spondyloarthritis and axial spondyloarthritis features. *Best estimate. HLA, human leukocyte antigen; LR, likelihood ratio; NSAID, nonsteroidal anti-inflammatory drug; SpA, spondyloarthritis; STIR, short tau inversion recovery. Reproduced with permission from © BMJ Publishing Group Ltd. 2013, Rudwaleit et al [11]. All Rights Reserved.

clinical parameter, but it is not essential. Also of note, CRP has only a limited value in a diagnostic approach because of a relatively low sensitivity and even in a patient with active disease a positive CRP can be found in only about 60%.

Screening for axial spondyloarthritis among patients with chronic back pain

In addition to establishing criteria for the classification and diagnosis of AS, screening strategies are of similar importance in alerting the primary care physician to a diagnosis of inflammatory spine disease in patients with chronic back pain and when to refer these patients to the rheumatologist for a final diagnosis. Whether chronic back pain patients are first seen by primary care physicians, orthopedists, physiotherapists, or other doctors varies from country to country. Therefore, such strategies have to be adapted to the local conditions. Recently, we have proposed screening parameters for early referral of AS patients by primary care physicians that are easy to apply [14]. Such parameters have to be

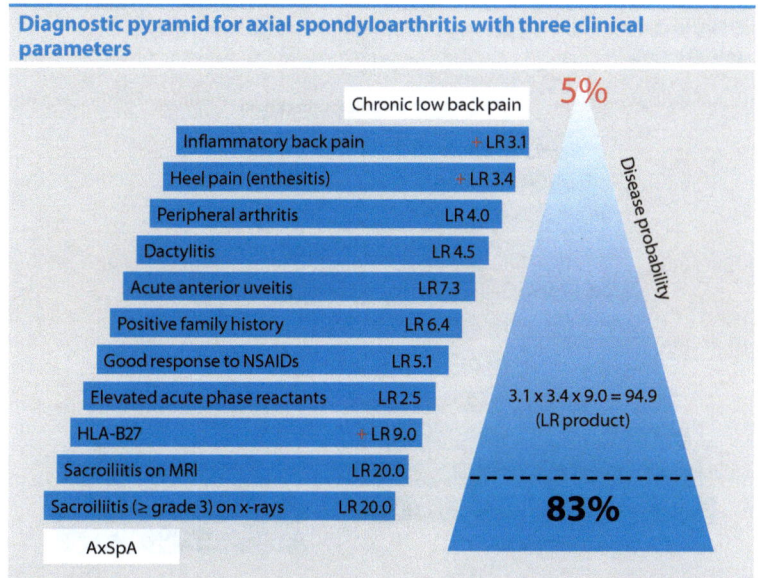

Figure 4.13 Diagnostic pyramid for axial spondyloarthritis with three clinical parameters. axSpA, axial spondyloarthritis; HLA, human leukocyte antigen; LR, likelihood ratio; NSAID, nonsteroidal anti-inflammatory drugs; pos, positive. Reproduced with permission from © John Wiley and Sons 2013, Rudwaleit et al [6]. All Rights Reserved.

relatively sensitive and specific for the disease studied, easy to apply by non-specialists and should not be too expensive. We performed a study in the environs of Berlin, Germany, asking all orthopedists and primary care physicians to refer to an early axSpA clinic patients with chronic back pain lasting for more than 3 months in whom the symptoms started at an age younger than 45, who fulfilled one or more of the following criteria: either fulfilling the clinical symptom of inflammatory back pain or being positive for HLA-B27, or showing evidence of sacroiliitis on imaging (Figure 4.15) [14]. Analysis of 350 referred patients showed that a final diagnosis of axSpA could be made in about 45% of patients (Figure 4.16), half of whom had nonradiographic sacroiliitis [15].

It could be confirmed in a multicenter study in Germany [16] and in another international multicenter study [17] that such an approach is indeed manageable and effective. Other approaches, using the clinical symptom of inflammatory back as referral parameter alone, have also been successfully applied and are summarized in a recent review [18].

Diagnostic pyramid for axial spondyloarthritis with four clinical parameters

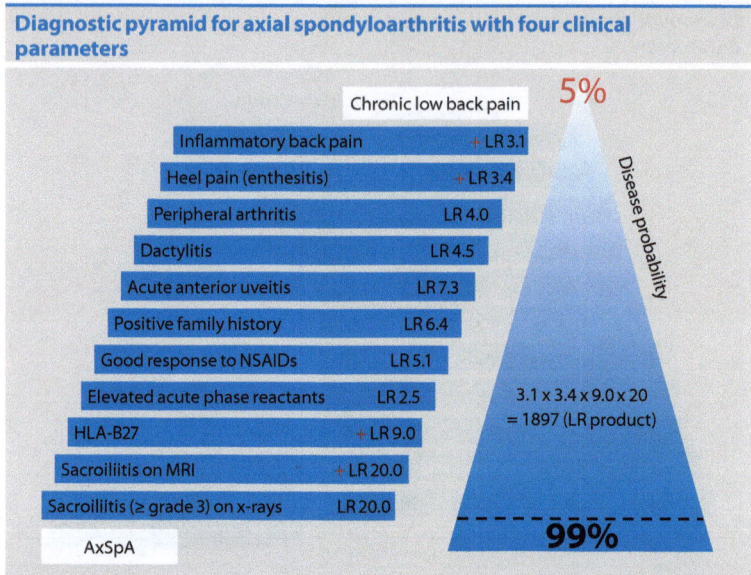

Figure 4.14 Diagnostic pyramid for axial spondyloarthritis with four clinical parameters.
axSpA, axial spondyloarthritis; HLA, human leukocyte antigen; LR, likelihood ratio; NSAID, nonsteroidal anti-inflammatory drugs; pos, positive. Reproduced with permission from © John Wiley and Sons 2013, Rudwaleit et al [6]. All Rights Reserved.

Possible screening approach for axial spondyloarthritis among patients with chronic lower back pain

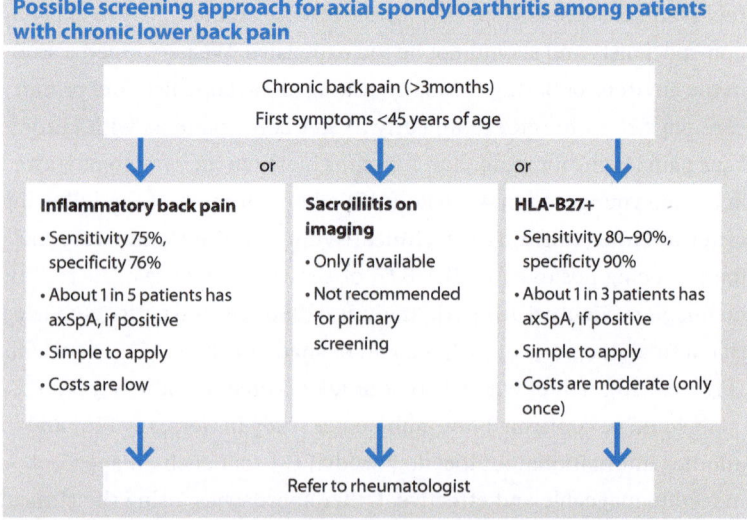

Figure 4.15 Possible screening approach for axial spondyloarthritis among patients with chronic lower back pain. axSpA, axial spondyloarthritis; HLA, human leukocyte antigen. Reproduced with permission from © BMJ Publishing Group Ltd. 2013, Sieper and Rudwaleit [14]. All Rights Reserved.

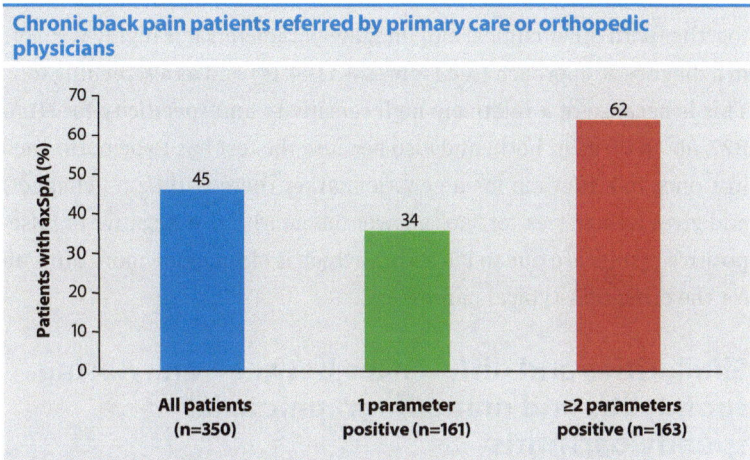

Figure 4.16 Chronic back pain patients referred by primary care or orthopedic physicians. axSpA, axial spondyloarthritis. Reproduced with permission from © BMJ Publishing Group Ltd. 2013, Brandt et al [15]. All Rights Reserved.

A most recent study resulted in a proposal for a two-step strategy: a chronic back pain patient seen in primary care should be referred to a rheumatologist if two out of three clinical parameters are positive (both sided buttock pain, improvement of chronic back pain by movement or psoriasis); if they are negative, HLA-B27 testing should be done and patients referred in case of a positive test [19]. These data clearly indicate that such a screening approach is feasible and effective, and that patients with nonradiographic axSpA (nr-axSpA) constitute a substantial part of the whole group of patients with axSpA.

The value of HLA-B27 for screening and diagnosis of axial spondyloarthritis

According to our calculations, a final diagnosis of axSpA can be made in one of three patients with chronic back pain (33%) who are positive for HLA-B27 [6,14]. This implies that two of three patients do not have this diagnosis despite being positive for HLA-B27! This figure was also confirmed in a recent study [15]. In the past, many patients with back pain have been labeled as having AS, simply because they are positive for HLA-B27 and consequently many rheumatologists have been reluctant to use HLA-B27 in a diagnostic approach. However, if HLA-B27 is used together with other clinical and imaging parameters it is highly valuable in a diagnostic approach (see Figures 4.11–4.14) and as a screening tool. This is because of a relatively high sensitivity and specificity for HLA-B27, about 90% for both, and also because the test has to be performed just once in a lifetime (as a genetic marker there will be no change!) and gives a clear "yes" or "no" answer (about 5% false-negative or false-positive results are due to lab error), which is often much more difficult for the other SpA-typical parameters.

Similarities and differences between ankylosing spondylitis and nonradiographic axial spondyloarthritis

Similarities and differences between the two subgroups have been described [20]. While they are similar in their clinical presentation, level of clinical disease activity, and response to tumor necrosis factor-blockade in patients with the same disease activity levels, they differ in their extent of structural damage (by definition), level of objective inflammation, as shown by the CRP values and MRI findings, and sex distribution [21,22]. Nr-axSpA patients have lower CRP-levels and more females are affected than in AS. Both elevated CRP and male gender have been known to be predictors of radiographic progression to AS, therefore probably explaining the higher prevalence of these factors in patients with AS.

References

1   van der Linden S, Valkenburg HA, Cats A. Evaluation of diagnostic criteria for ankylosing spondylitis. A proposal for modification of the New York criteria. *Arthritis Rheum.* 1984;27:361-368.

2   van der Linden SM, Valkenburg HA, de Jongh BM, Cats A. The risk of developing ankylosing spondylitis in HLA-B27 positive individuals. A comparison of relatives of spondylitis patients with the general population. *Arthritis Rheum.* 1984;27:241-249.

3   Bennett PH, Burch TA (eds.). Population studies of the rheumatic diseases. Amsterdam: Excerpta Medica Foundation, International Congress Series: 1966,148: 456-457.

4   Feldtkeller E, Bruckel J, Khan MA. Scientific contributions of ankylosing spondylitis patient advocacy groups. *Curr Opin Rheumatol.* 2000;12:239-247.

5   Dougados M, van der Linden S, et al. The European Spondylarthropathy Study Group preliminary criteria for the classification of spondylarthropathy. *Arthritis Rheum.* 1991;34:1218-1227.

6   Rudwaleit M, Khan MA, Sieper J. The challenge of diagnosis and classification in early ankylosing spondylitis: do we need new criteria? *Arthritis Rheum.* 2005;52:1000-1008.

7 Rudwaleit M, Jurik AG, Hermann KG, et al. Defining active sacroiliitis on magnetic resonance imaging (MRI) for classification of axial spondyloarthritis: a consensual approach by the ASAS/OMERACT MRI group. *Ann Rheum Dis.* 2009;68:1520-1527.

8 Braun J, Bollow M, Eggens U, König H, Distler A, Sieper J. Use of dynamic magnetic resonance imaging with fast imaging in the detection of early and advanced sacroiliitis in spondylarthropathy patients. *Arthritis Rheum.* 1994;37:1039-1045.

9 Bennett AN, McGonagle D, O'Connor P, et al. Severity of baseline magnetic resonance imaging-evident sacroiliitis and HLA-B27 status in early inflammatory back pain predict radiographically evident ankylosing spondylitis at eight years. *Arthritis Rheum.* 2008;58:3413-3418.

10 Rudwaleit M, van der Heijde D, Landewé R, et al. The development of Assessment of SpondyloArthritis international Society (ASAS) classification criteria for axial spondyloarthritis (part II): validation and final selection. *Ann Rheum Dis.* 2009;68:777-783.

11 Rudwaleit M, van der Heijde D, Khan MA, Braun J, Sieper J. How to diagnose axial spondyloarthritis early. *Ann Rheum Dis.* 2004;63:535-543.

12 van den Berg R, de Hooge M, Rudwaleit M, et al. ASAS modification of the Berlin algorithm for diagnosing axial spondyloarthritis: results from the SPondyloArthritis Caught Early (SPACE)-cohort and from the Assessment of SpondyloArthritis international Society (ASAS)-cohort. *Ann Rheum Dis.* 2013;72:1646-1653.

13 Underwood MR, Dawes P. Inflammatory back pain in primary care. *Br J Rheumatol.* 1995;34:1074-1077.

14 Sieper J, Rudwaleit M. Early referral recommendations for ankylosing spondylitis (including pre-radiographic and radiographic forms) in primary care. *Ann Rheum Dis.* 2005;64:659-663.

15 Brandt HC, Spiller I, Song IH, Vahldiek JL, Rudwaleit M, Sieper J. Performance of referral recommendations in patients with chronic back pain and suspected axial spondyloarthritis. *Ann Rheum Dis.* 2007;66:1479-1484.

16 Poddubnyy D, Vahldiek J, Spiller I, et al. Evaluation of 2 screening strategies for early identification of patients with axial spondyloarthritis in primary care. *J Rheumatol.* 2011;38:2452-2460.

17 Sieper J, Srinivasan S, Zamani O, et al. Comparison of two referral strategies for diagnosis of axial spondyloarthritis: the Recognising and Diagnosing Ankylosing Spondylitis Reliably (RADAR) study. *Ann Rheum Dis.* 2012;72:1621-1627.

18 Rudwaleit M, Sieper J. Referral strategies for early diagnosis of axial spondyloarthritis. *Nat Rev Rheumatol.* 2012;8:262-268.

19 Braun A, Gnann H, Saracbasi E, et al. Optimizing the identification of patients with axial spondyloarthritis in primary care--the case for a two-step strategy combining the most relevant clinical items with HLA B27. *Rheumatology (Oxford).* 2013;52:1418-1424.

20 Sieper J, van der Heijde D. Review: Nonradiographic axial spondyloarthritis: new definition of an old disease? *Arthritis Rheum.* 2013;65:543-551.

21 Rudwaleit M, Haibel H, Baraliakos X, et al. The early disease stage in axial spondylarthritis: results from the German Spondyloarthritis Inception Cohort. *Arthritis Rheum.* 2009;60:721-727.

22 Kiltz U, Baraliakos X, Karakostas P, et al. Do patients with non-radiographic axial spondylarthritis differ from patients with ankylosing spondylitis? *Arthritis Care Res (Hoboken).* 2012;64:1415-1422.

Chapter 5

Imaging in axial spondyloarthritis

Radiographs and magnetic resonance imaging (MRI) for sacroiliac (SI) joints and the spine are the most important imaging techniques for the diagnosis and follow-up of patients with spondyloarthritis (SpA), including response to treatment. If other sites outside the axial skeleton are affected they can also be investigated by these methods. In general, radiographs should not be performed more frequently than every 2 years because (chronic) changes occur slowly and investigations with MRI can be used more frequently, according to the clinical situation.

Radiographs

The investigation of SI joints and the spine by radiographs has been used since the 1930s for the diagnosis and staging of patients with ankylosing spondylitis (AS). In contrast to MRI, radiographs can detect only chronic bony changes (damage) that are the consequence of inflammation and not inflammation itself. Therefore, radiographs are not suitable for early diagnosis of SpA, although they are still the method of choice for the detection of chronic changes and are widely used for diagnostic purposes in patients with already established disease (see modified New York criteria in Chapter 4). Erosive bony changes can also be detected early in the course of the disease by radiographs, although other methods, such as computed tomography (CT) and MRI, are superior for this. Radiographs are most important for the detection and follow-up of new bone formation, such as syndesmophytes in the spine.

J. Sieper and J. Braun, *Clinician's Manual on Axial Spondyloarthritis*,
DOI: 10.1007/978-1-907673-85-6_5, © Springer Healthcare 2014

SI changes can be scored according to the grading discussed earlier in Chapter 4, which also shows examples of various grades of sacroiliitis (see Figures 4.3–4.5). Different approaches have been proposed for the radiological investigation of the SI joints with the intention of getting an optimal view of this irregularly shaped joint. None of them has been shown to be clearly superior. The Assessment in SpondyloArthritis international Society (ASAS) recommends performing radiographs of the whole pelvis because this allows assessment of the hip joints, as well as the SI joints; the hip joints are relatively frequently affected in SpA. One possible differential diagnosis, osteitis condensans ilii, which can be found preferentially in middle-aged women, is shown in Figure 5.1.

When investigating the spine by radiographs, the cervical and lumbar spine should be included. Although changes in the thoracic spine are frequent, they are more difficult to detect because of the overlying lung tissue, so radiographs of the thoracic spine are not routinely assessed. Figure 5.2 shows typical spinal lesions that can be seen on radiographs: squaring of the vertebral body as a result of remodeling due to inflammation and new bone formation, sclerosis of the vertebral edges as a consequence of inflammation (shiny corners) and syndesmophytes [1]. Syndesmophytes typically grow in a vertical direction whereas spondylophytes – typical for degenerative spine disease – grow in a

Osteitis condensans ilii

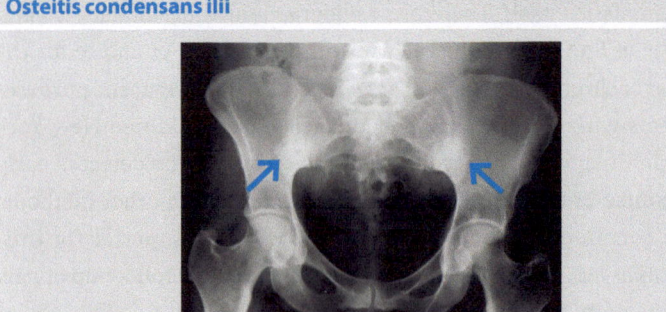

Figure 5.1 Osteitis condensans ilii. Radiograph of a woman aged 45 years with osteitis condensans ilii. The patient had low back pain for 3 months and was negative for human leukocyte antigen (HLA)-B27. Reproduced with permission from © ASAS [www.asas-group.org]. All Rights Reserved.

horizontal direction (Figure 5.3) [1]. Figure 5.4 shows an example of an already ankylosed facet joint in a patient with AS. Figure 5.5 shows a patient with AS with an Andersson II lesion (CT scan) resulting from a preceding spondylodiscitis with a subsequent insufficiency fracture at this site [2]. Of note, osteoporosis of the spine as a consequence of local and systemic inflammation occurs more often in patients with AS compared with age-matched controls, with increased risk for vertebral fractures, but not for nonvertebral fractures [3].

Figure 5.6 shows a radiograph from a patient with diffuse idiopathic skeletal hyperostosis (DISH; also known as Forestier disease), an important differential diagnosis of advanced AS. Note that the ligament in front of the vertebrae is ossified in combination with severe degenerative spinal changes, in the absence of AS-typical syndesmophytes. Radiographs of

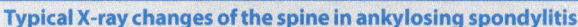

Typical X-ray changes of the spine in ankylosing spondylitis

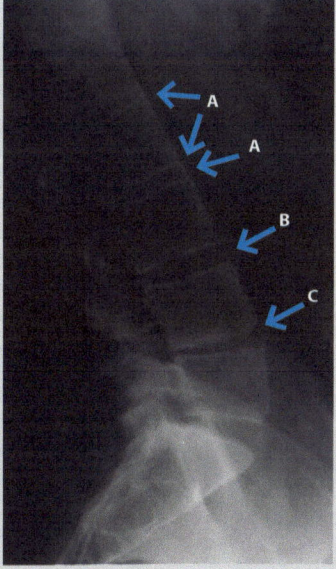

Figure 5.2 Typical X-ray changes of the spine in ankylosing spondylitis. A, bridging syndesmophytes; **B,** small syndesmophyte; **C,** erosion and sclerosis. Reproduced with permission from © BMJ Publishing Group Ltd. 2013, Baraliakos et al [1]. All Rights Reserved.

X-ray of a spine with spondylophytes in degenerative spine disease

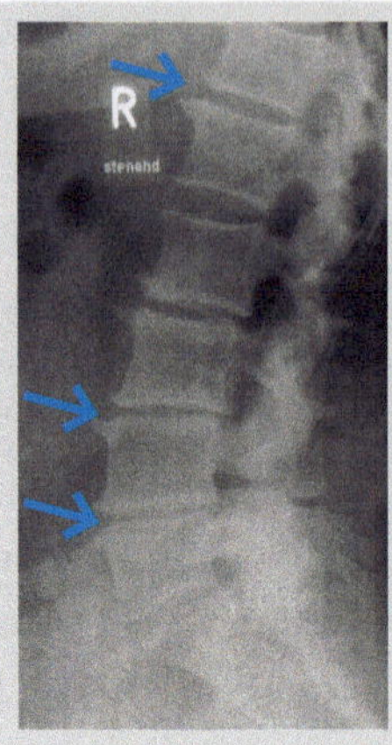

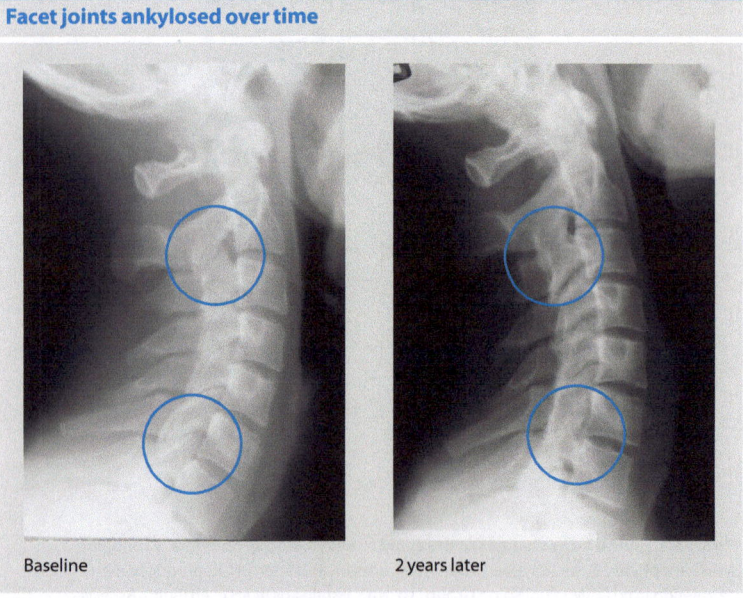

Figure 5.3 X-ray of a spine with spondylophytes in degenerative spine disease.
Spondylophytes (arrows) are typical for degenerative spine disease and have a horizontal growth, while syndesmophytes (not shown here) show a vertical growth.

Facet joints ankylosed over time

Baseline

2 years later

Figure 5.4 Facet joints ankylosed over time.

Computed tomography image showing Andersson II lesion in ankylosing spondylitis

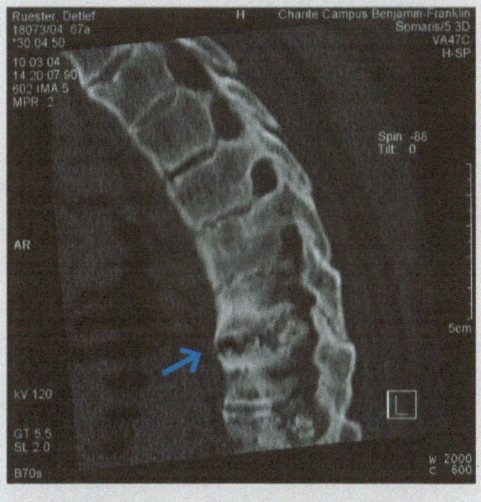

Figure 5.5 Computed tomography image showing Andersson II lesion in ankylosing spondylitis. Spondylodiscitis with insufficiency fracture. Reproduced with permission from © Sieper 2013 [2]. All Rights Reserved.

the SI joints are mostly normal although ossification of ligaments can imitate ankylosed SI joints.

Magnetic resonance imaging

MRI studies of the SI joints and the spine in patients with SpA have made a major contribution in the last decade to a better understanding of the course of the disease, early diagnosis, and use as an objective outcome measure for clinical trials.

Active inflammatory changes are best visualized by a fat-saturated, T2-weighted, turbo spin-echo sequence, or a short tau inversion recovery (STIR) sequence with a high resolution that detects even minor fluid collections, such as bone marrow edema. Without fat saturation, fluid accumulation cannot be differentiated from fatty degeneration using this technique. Alternatively, administration of a paramagnetic contrast medium (gadolinium) detects increased perfusion (osteitis) in a T1-weighted sequence with fat saturation. These two sequences

Diffuse idiopathic skeletal hyperostosis

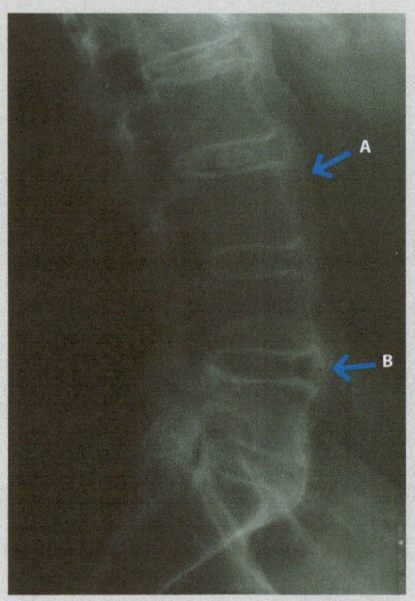

Figure 5.6 Diffuse idiopathic skeletal hyperostosis. Radiograph of a male patient aged 75 years with diffuse idiopathic skeletal hyperostosis who experienced chronic back pain. **A,** ossification of ligament and no syndesmophytes; **B,** spondylophytes.

give largely overlapping information, although occasionally applying both methods can give additional value. Chronic changes, such as fatty degeneration and erosions, are best seen using a T1-weighted, turbo spin-echo sequence.

The SI joints are imaged by MRI using a semicoronal section orientation along the long axis of the sacral bone. A positive MRI (active inflammatory lesions) of the SI joints, also used in the ASAS classification criteria for axial SpA (axSpA) [4], is defined as the presence of definite subchondral bone marrow edema/osteitis highly suggestive of sacroiliitis [5]. A typical example of an active sacroiliitis with subchondral bone marrow edema is shown in Figure 5.7. If there is only one signal (lesion), this should be present on at least two slices. If there is more than one signal on a single slice, one slice may be enough. The presence of just synovitis, capsulitis, or enthesitis with no concomitant

Active inflammatory sacroiliitis of the right joint by MRI

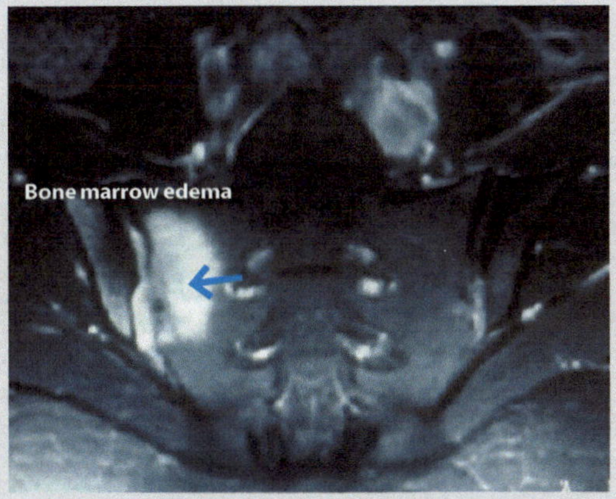

Figure 5.7 Active inflammatory sacroiliitis of the right joint by MRI.

subchondral bone marrow edema/osteitis is compatible with sacroiliitis but not sufficient to make a diagnosis of active sacroiliitis [6]. Possible differential diagnoses for an active inflammatory sacroiliitis in SpA are infectious sacroiliitis (typically also affecting the surrounding soft tissue), fracture of the ileum bone or the sacrum bone, and bone tumor. T1-weighted sequences can detect chronic changes, such as erosions and fatty degeneration, which are early signs of chronic damage (Figure 5.8).

An efficient spinal imaging protocol comprises a sagittal, T1-weighted, turbo spin-echo sequence and a sagittal, fat-saturated, T2-weighted turbo spin-echo or STIR sequence with high resolution. Coronal slices of the entire spine may be used for better assessment of the costover-tebral and costotransverse joints and the facet joints. Some examples of active inflammation of the spine in patients with axSpA are shown in the following figures: spondylitis anterior (Figure 5.9), spondylitis posterior (Figure 5.10), and spondylodiscitis (Figure 5.11) [7]. A positive spinal MRI for inflammation was defined by ASAS as the presence of anterior/posterior spondylitis in ≥3 sites. Evidence of fatty deposition at several vertebral corners was found to be suggestive of axSpA, especially in younger adults [8]. However, active inflammation of the spine is not part of the current ASAS classification criteria for axSpA.

MRI showing a patient with chronic sacroiliitis

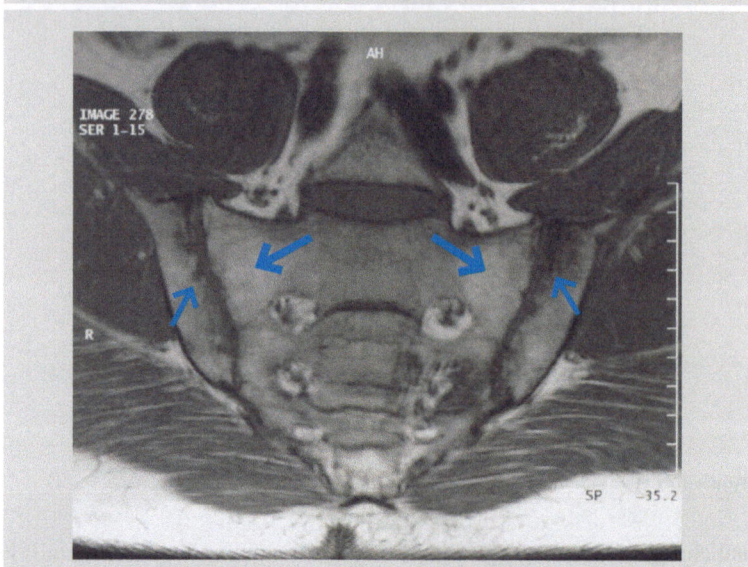

Figure 5.8 MRI showing a patient with chronic sacroiliitis. Erosions (arrows) and fatty degeneration (bold arrows). T1-sequence.

An important and sometimes difficult differential diagnosis is erosive osteochondritis (Figure 5.12) as a consequence of degenerative disc disease, which resembles the spondylodiscitis seen in patients with SpA. These lesions are most often located in the lumbar spine and patients would normally have no other features typical for AS/SpA and normal SI joints. T1-weighted sequences can also detect chronic changes, such as erosions and fatty degeneration – similar to the SI joints – in the spine of patients with axSpA.

Other imaging techniques

Scintigraphy has been used for many decades for the detection of active inflammation in patients with SpA. However, it no longer plays a role in the diagnosis and management of patients with SpA because of limited sensitivity and specificity and has been replaced by MRI [9]. Chronic bony changes can be better detected by CT (Figure 5.13) rather than radiographs. However, CT is rarely used because of a much higher

Spondylitis anterior by MRI

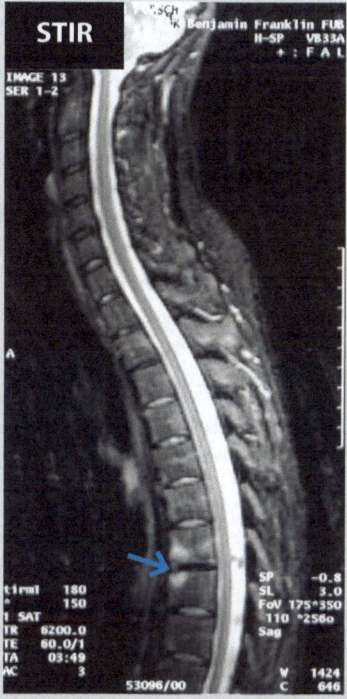

Figure 5.9 Spondylitis anterior by MRI. Spondylitis anterior (arrow) with active inflammation. STIR, short tau inversion recovery.

Active spondylitis posterior by MRI

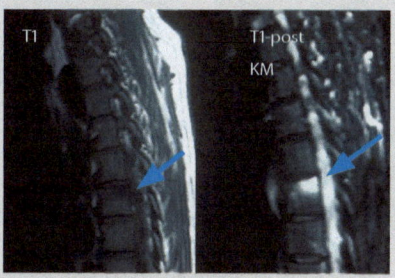

Figure 5.10 Active spondylitis posterior by MRI. Reproduced with permission from © Elsevier Limited 2013, Braun et al [7]. All Rights Reserved.

Spondylodiscitis by MRI in axial spondyloarthritis

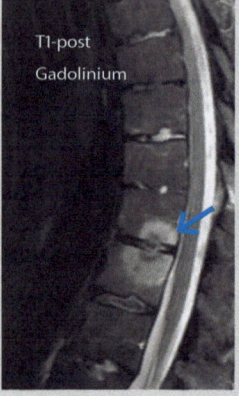

Figure 5.11 Spondylodiscitis by MRI in axial spondyloarthritis. Reproduced with permission from © KG Hermann, Berlin, Germany. All Rights Reserved.

Erosive osteochondrosis with bone marrow edema

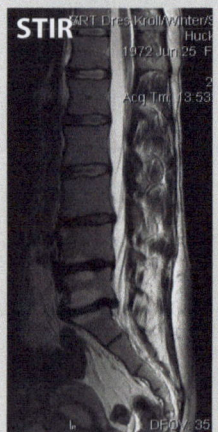 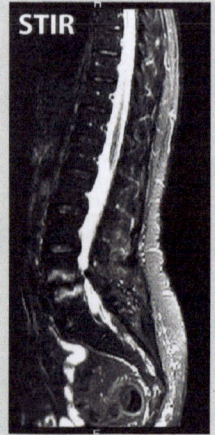

Figure 5.12 Erosive osteochondrosis with bone marrow edema. A, early case with edema but without major erosions; **B,** more advanced case with edema and erosions. STIR, short tau inversion recovery.

Sacroiliitis grade II bilaterally on computed tomography

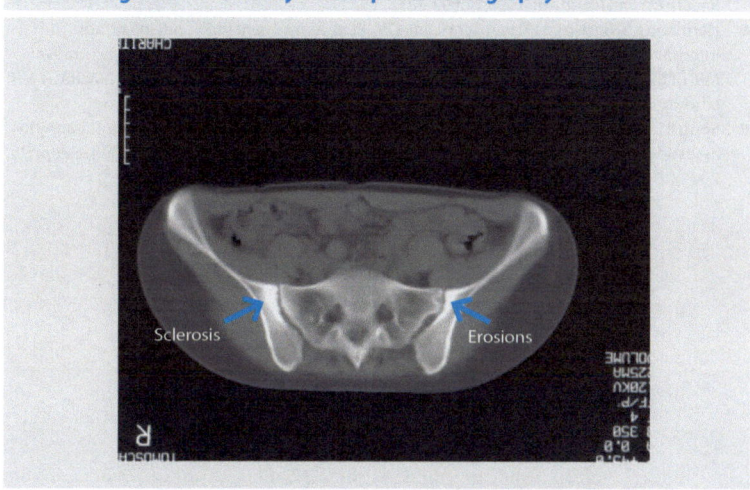

Figure 5.13 Sacroiliitis grade II bilaterally on computed tomography.

radiation exposure. Active inflammatory changes cannot be seen by CT and fatty degeneration of the bone marrow, as an early sign of chronic change, is detectable only by MRI and not by CT.

For a more detailed description of imaging in AS, including its early forms, see also the ASAS handbook on assessment of spondyloarthritis [6].

References

1   Baraliakos X, Listing J, Rudwaleit M, Brandt J, Sieper J, Braun J. Radiographic progression in patients with ankylosing spondylitis after 2 years of treatment with the tumour necrosis factor alpha antibody infliximab. *Ann Rheum Dis*. 2005;64:1462-1466.

2   Sieper J. Management of ankylosing spondylitis. In: *Rheumatology*, 4th edition. Edited by MC Hochberg, AJ Silman, et al. London: Mosby, 2008;1159.

3   Vosse D, Landewé R, van der Heijde D, van der Linden S, van Staa TP, Geusens P. Ankylosing spondylitis and the risk of fracture: results from a large primary care-based nested case-control study. *Ann Rheum Dis*. 2009;68:1839-1842.

4   Rudwaleit M, van der Heijde D, Landewé R, et al. The development of Assessment of SpondyloArthritis international Society classification criteria for axial spondyloarthritis (part II): validation and final selection. *Ann Rheum Dis*. 2009;68:777-783.

5   Rudwaleit M, Jurik AG, Hermann KG, et al. Defining active sacroiliitis on magnetic resonance imaging (MRI) for classification of axial spondyloarthritis: a consensual approach by the ASAS/OMERACT MRI group. *Ann Rheum Dis*. 2009;68:1520-1527.

6   Sieper J, Rudwaleit M, Baraliakos X, et al. The Assessment of SpondyloArthritis international Society (ASAS) handbook: a guide to assess spondyloarthritis. *Ann Rheum Dis*. 2009;68 (Suppl 2):ii1-44.

7 Braun J, Bollow M, Sieper J. Radiologic diagnosis and pathology of the spondyloarthropathies. *Rheum Dis Clin North Am.* 1998;24:697-735.

8 Hermann KG, Baraliakos X, van der Heijde DM, et al; Assessment in SpondyloArthritis international Society (ASAS). Descriptions of spinal MRI lesions and definition of a positive MRI of the spine in axial spondyloarthritis: a consensual approach by the ASAS/OMERACT MRI study group. *Ann Rheum Dis.* 2012;71:1278-1288.

9 Song IH, Carrasco-Fernández J, Rudwaleit M, Sieper J. The diagnostic value of scintigraphy in assessing sacroiliitis in ankylosing spondylitis: a systematic literature research. *Ann Rheum Dis.* 2008;67:1535-1540.

Chapter 6

Management of axial spondyloarthritis

Recently, the Assessment of SpondyloArthritis international Society (ASAS) and European League Against Rheumatism (EULAR) recommendations on the management of ankylosing spondylitis (AS) were updated, based on a thorough analysis of the available literature and on a meeting of spondyloarthritis (SpA) experts. These recommendations are shown in Figures 6.1 and 6.2 [1]. Nondrug approaches are part of the therapy

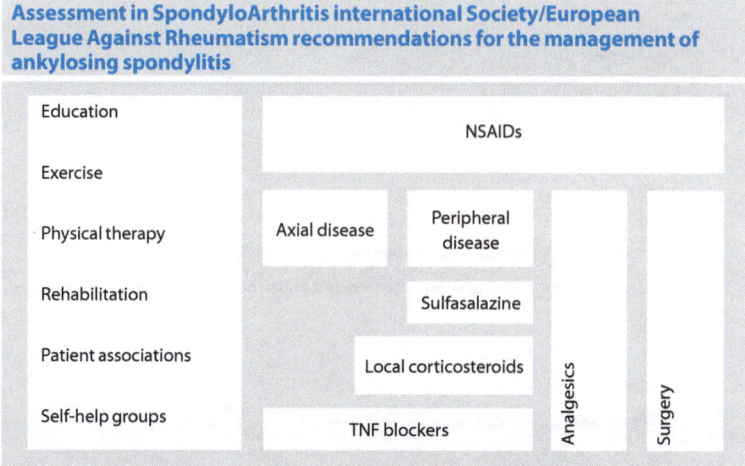

Figure 6.1 Assessment in SpondyloArthritis international Society/European League Against Rheumatism recommendations for the management of ankylosing spondylitis. NSAID, nonsteroidal anti-inflammatory drugs; TNF, tumor necrosis factor. Adapted from Braun et al [1].

J. Sieper and J. Braun, *Clinician's Manual on Axial Spondyloarthritis*, DOI: 10.1007/978-1-907673-85-6_6, © Springer Healthcare 2014

Assessment in SpondyloArthritis international Society/European League Against Rheumatism recommendations for the management of ankylosing spondylitis (continues over)

The overarching principles of the management of patients with AS are:

AS is a potentially severe disease with diverse manifestations, usually requiring multidisciplinary treatment coordinated by the rheumatologist.

The primary goal of treating the patient with AS is to maximize long term health-related quality of life through control of symptoms and

Inflammation, prevention of progressive structural damage, preservation/normalization of function and social participation.

Treatment of AS should aim at the best care and must be based on a shared decision between the patient and the rheumatologist.

The optimal management of patients with AS requires a combination of nonpharmacological and pharmacological treatment modalities.

1. General treatment

The treatment of patients with AS should be tailored according to:

The current manifestations of the disease (axial, peripheral, entheseal, extraarticular symptoms, and signs).

The level of current symptoms, clinical findings, and prognostic indicators.

The general clinical status (age, gender, comorbidity, concomitant medications, psychosocial factors).

2. Disease monitoring

The disease monitoring of patients with AS should include:

Patient history (eg, questionnaires)

Clinical parameters

Laboratory tests

Imaging

All according to the clinical presentation as well as the ASAS core set

The frequency of monitoring should be decided on an individual basis depending on:

Course of symptoms

Severity

Treatment

3. Nonpharmacological treatment

The cornerstone of nonpharmacological treatment of patients with AS is patient education and regular exercise.

Figure 6.2 Assessment in SpondyloArthritis international Society/European League Against Rheumatism recommendations for the management of ankylosing spondylitis (continues over).

Assessment in SpondyloArthritis international Society/European League Against Rheumatism recommendations for the management of ankylosing spondylitis (continues overleaf)

3. Nonpharmacological treatment (continued)

Home exercises are effective. Physical therapy with supervised exercises, land or water based, individually or in a group, should be preferred as these are more effective than home exercises.

Patient associations and self-help groups may be useful.

4. Extraarticular manifestations and comorbidities

The frequently observed extraarticular manifestations, for example, psoriasis, uveitis, and IBD, should be managed in collaboration with the respective specialists.

Rheumatologists should be aware of the increased risk of cardiovascular disease and osteoporosis.

5. Nonsteroidal anti-inflammatory drugs

NSAIDs, including Coxibs, are recommended as first-line drug treatment for patients with AS with pain and stiffness.

Continuous treatment with NSAIDs is preferred for patients with persistently active, symptomatic disease.

Cardiovascular, gastrointestinal, and renal risks should be taken into account when prescribing NSAIDs.

6. Analgesics

Analgesics, such as paracetamol and opioid (like) drugs, might be considered for residual pain after previously recommended treatments have failed, are contraindicated, and/or poorly tolerated.

7. Glucocorticoids

Corticosteroid injections directed to the local site of musculoskeletal inflammation may be considered.

The use of systemic glucocorticoids for axial disease is not supported by evidence.

8. Disease-modifying antirheumatic drugs

There is no evidence for the efficacy of DMARD, including sulfasalazine and methotrexate, for the treatment of axial disease.

Sulfasalazine may be considered in patients with peripheral arthritis.

9. Anti-tumor necrosis factor therapy

Anti-TNF therapy should be given to patients with persistently high disease activity despite conventional treatments, according to the ASAS recommendations.

There is no evidence to support the obligatory use of DMARD before or concomitant with anti-TNF therapy in patients with axial disease.

Figure 6.2 Assessment in SpondyloArthritis international Society/European League Against Rheumatism recommendations for the management of ankylosing spondylitis (continues overleaf).

Assessment in SpondyloArthritis international Society/European League Against Rheumatism recommendations for the management of ankylosing spondylitis (continued)

9. Anti-tumor necrosis factor therapy (contined)

There is no evidence to support a difference in efficacy of the various TNF inhibitors on the axial and articular/entheseal disease manifestations; but in the presence of IBD a difference in gastrointestinal efficacy needs to be taken into account.

Switching to a second TNF blocker might be beneficial especially in patients with loss of response.

There is no evidence to support the use of biological agents other than TNF inhibitors in AS.

10. Surgery

Total hip arthroplasty should be considered in patients with refractory pain or disability and radiographic evidence of structural damage, independent of age.

Spinal corrective osteotomy may be considered in patients with severe disabling deformity.

In patients with AS and an acute vertebral fracture a spinal surgeon should be consulted.

11. Changes in the disease course

If a significant change in the course of the disease occurs, other causes than inflammation, such as a spinal fracture, should be considered and appropriate evaluation, including imaging, should be performed.

Figure 6.2 Assessment in SpondyloArthritis international Society/European League Against Rheumatism recommendations for the management of ankylosing spondylitis (continued). AS, ankylosing spondylitis; ASAS, Assessment in SpondyloArthritis international Society; DMARD, disease-modifying antirheumatic drugs; IBD, inflammatory bowel disease; NSAID, nonsteroidal anti-inflammatory drugs; TNF, tumor necrosis factor. Reproduced with permission from ©BMJ Publishing Group Ltd. 2013, Braun et al [1]. All Rights Reserved.

at all stages of the disease. For the predominantly axial manifestation, the treatment options are limited to nonsteroidal anti-inflammatory drugs (NSAID) as a kind of basic treatment, followed by tumor necrosis factor (TNF)-blocker therapy if this conventional treatment fails. If the clinical picture is dominated by peripheral symptoms, such as arthritis or enthesitis, treatment with sulfasalazine and/or local steroid injection should be tried first before TNF blockers are considered.

Nondrug treatment

Physiotherapy is the most important nonpharmacological aspect of AS management and was for a long time the most important form of management. Its primary aims are to prevent and/or reduce restriction of spinal mobility and the development of disability, and to improve the symptoms of pain and stiffness. Once the diagnosis has been made, the patient should be referred to a physical therapist who will teach the patient the exercises that he or she should perform regularly. As the main long-term outcome flexion deformity of the spine should be prevented; therefore, exercises concentrate on extension and rotation of the spine. An exercise sequence for patients with AS is shown in Figure 6.3.

Patients should be advised to exercise daily at home and to attend weekly group physical therapy. The patient's own efforts are the key to future success and the patient with AS has to be convinced that a daily exercise program should become a normal part of the day. In the long-term, many patients do not need regular prescriptions; however, there should be some mechanisms in place to ensure that the patient is seen and assessed regularly by the physical therapist. If patients are symptomatic and complain about pain or stiffness, they should be treated in addition with NSAIDs (see below) or other effective drugs to permit full mobilization during the exercises. These exercises should be continued regularly and lifelong. Furthermore, patients should be encouraged to participate in moderate sport activities, such as swimming and cycling.

Patient education is an essential part of nonpharmacological therapy and should include information about pathogenesis, clinical manifestations and course of the disease, physiotherapy and ergotherapy, how to cope with the disease, and counseling about the socioeconomic consequences of the disease. Patients should also be encouraged to get engaged in patient associations and patient self-help groups.

Drug treatment options
Nonsteroidal anti-inflammatory drug treatment
The NSAIDs are still regarded as the cornerstone of pharmacological intervention for AS with a good anti-inflammatory capacity, reducing pain and stiffness rapidly after 48–72 hours [2,3]. Most patients with AS report a good or very good efficacy when treated with a full dose of an NSAID, in contrast to patients with chronic back pain from other causes (Figure 6.4) [4]. Figure 6.5 shows NSAIDs that are used for the treatment of AS [3]. The dosing should be adjusted to the clinical symptoms and the half-life of the drug: normally the effect of the drug should

Physical therapy for patients with ankylosing spondylitis (continues over)

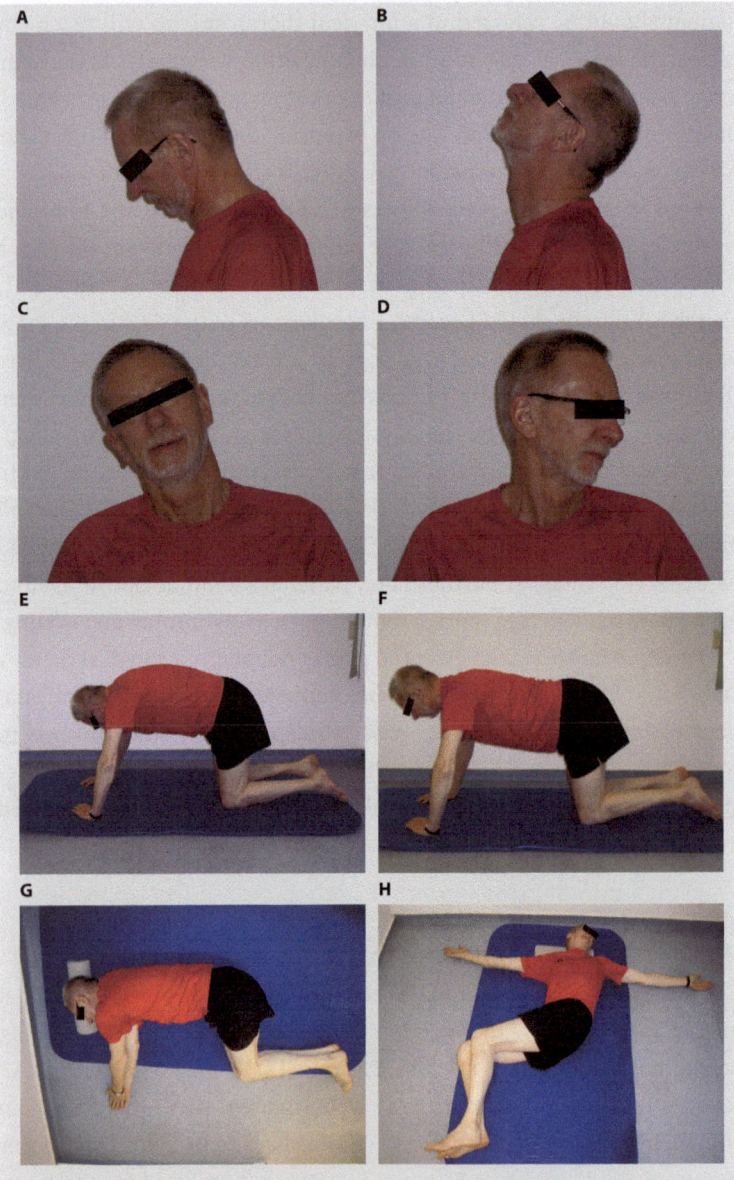

Figure 6.3 Physical therapy for patients with ankylosing spondylitis (continues over).
An exercise sequence used in ankylosing spondylitis. Cervical spine exercises include: **A,** full flexion; **B,** extension; **C,** lateral flexion; and, **D,** rotation. A sequence of, **E,** back flexion and, **F,** extension is followed by rotation in a lying position **(G, H)**.

Physical therapy for patients with ankylosing spondylitis (contined)

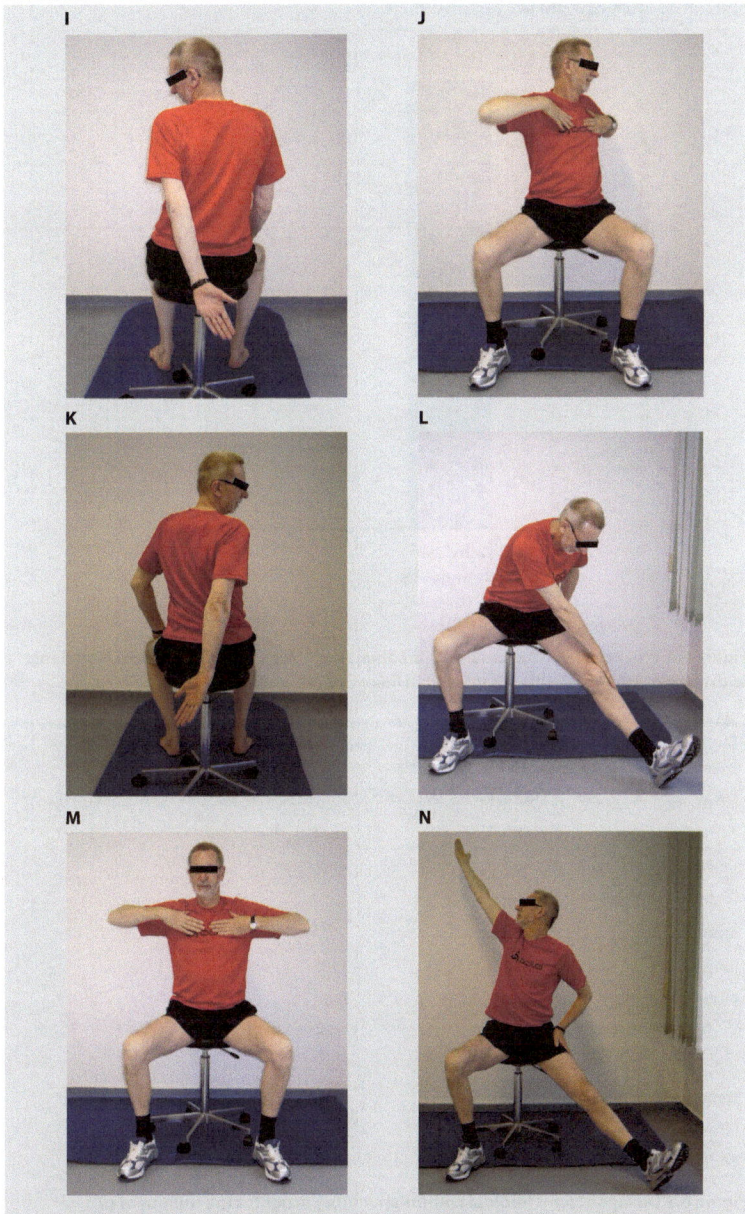

Figure 6.3 Physical therapy for patients with ankylosing spondylitis (continued).
A sequence of rotations in a sitting position, **I–N**. Finally, breathing is practiced using the
thoracic muscles (not shown).

Efficacy of nonsteroidal anti-inflammatory drugs for the treatment of patients with ankylosing spondylitis

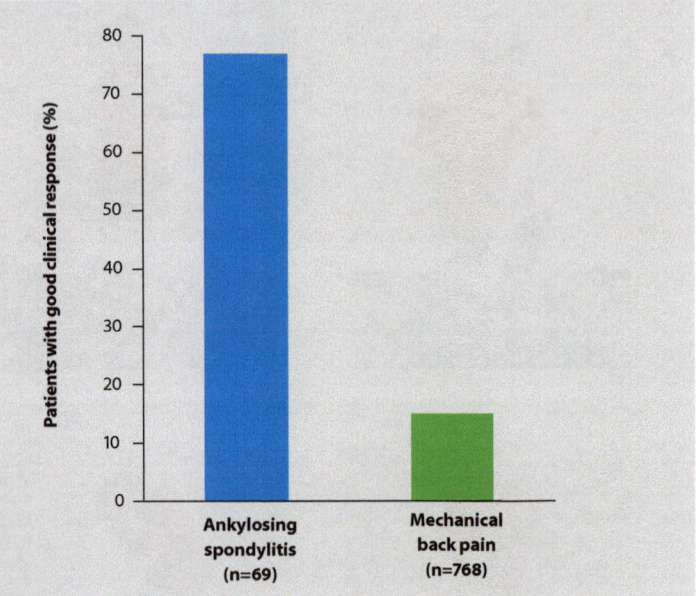

Figure 6.4 Efficacy of nonsteroidal anti-inflammatory drugs for the treatment of patients with ankylosing spondylitis. Adapted from Amor et al [4].

Dosage of nonsteroidal anti-inflammatory drugs for the treatment of patient with ankylosing spondylitis

Drug	Half-life (hours)	Approved maximum daily dosage (mg)†
Aceclofenac	about 4	200
Celecoxib	8–12	400
Diclofenac*	about 2	150
Etoricoxib	about 22	90
Ibuprofen	1.8–3.5	2400
Indomethacin*	about 2	150
Ketoprofen	1.5–2.5	200
Meloxicam	about 20	15
Naproxen	10–18	1000
Piroxicam	30–60	20
Phenylbutazone	50–100	600

Figure 6.5 Dosage of nonsteroidal anti-inflammatory drugs for the treatment of patient with ankylosing spondylitis. *Slow-release formula available; †Normally for arthritis. Reproduced with permission from © John Wiley and Sons 2013, Song et al [3]. All Rights Reserved.

cover the night and the early morning (ie, morning stiffness); however, often 24-hour treatment is necessary. Phenylbutazone, which has been approved for short-term treatment, is probably one of the most effective NSAIDs, but should be reserved for patients in whom other NSAIDs failed and should be given for only a few days because of possible bone marrow toxicity. At least two NSAIDs should be tested before NSAID treatment failure is assumed. A recent study in patients with early (symptom duration of <3 years) axial SpA (axSpA), including both patients with AS and nonradiologic axSpA (nr-axSpA), found a high remission rate of 33% in patients treated with a full dose of an NSAID over 6 months [5], indicating that patients early in the course of their disease might respond better to NSAIDs than later on.

Frequently patients are not treated with a full dose of NSAIDs and/or are not treated continuously despite being symptomatic. A major reason for this is that both patients and treating physicians are often concerned about the toxicity of continuous NSAID treatment [6]. We have recently summarized and discussed the benefits and risks of NSAID treatment in AS [3]; besides good efficacy for signs and symptoms there is even evidence that continuous therapy with NSAIDs might stop the new formation of syndesmophytes in the spine [7]. In two more recent studies it could be shown that especially C-reactive protein (CRP)-positive patients with AS benefit from a consequent NSAIDs treatment while there was no difference between low and high NSAIDs-treated patients in the CRP-negative groups [8,9]. A likely explanation for such an effect is by direct inhibition of osteoblast activity by NSAIDs, through the suppression of prostaglandins.

There are now sufficient data available on the risks of long-term treatment with NSAIDs in several large non-AS trials: the probability in patients younger than 60 years and with no gastrointestinal (GI) or cardiovascular (CV) comorbidities is 1% or less of developing serious GI or CV side effects when treated with a full dose of an NSAID for 1 year. Also the risk for renal and liver side effects is known and seems to be acceptable [3]. Thus, when patients with AS are active, they should be treated with a sufficient, and if necessary continuous, dose of NSAIDs. Nonetheless, the CV and GI risk is probably increased compared to a control population not treated with NSAIDs [10] and patients should be informed about and monitored for potential toxicity both before and during treatment. However, the vast majority of the side effect data for NSAIDs treatment has been raised in a non-AS population and a recent investigation found an increased mortality in patients with AS to be associated with an elevated CRP but also with not-using NSAIDs therapy [11]. Thus, more data on NSAIDs side effects specifically for the axSpA population is wanted.

Simple analgesics, such as paracetamol and opioids, have at most a limited role in the treatment of AS and are used in patients who have contraindications to treatment with NSAIDs and/or a TNF blocker.

Corticosteroids and disease-modifying antirheumatic drugs

There is no clear role for systemic corticosteroids in the treatment of AS because a high dose is normally necessary to achieve a measurable clinical improvement. Indeed, in a placebo-controlled trial over 2 weeks only treatment with 50 mg prednisolone per day was associated with a clinically relevant improvement of the disease activity in patients with AS compared to patients treated either with 20 mg/day or with placebo [12]. In case of inflammation at single joints, such as a sacroiliac (SI) joint or peripheral joint, local steroid injections have proved effective [13].

Conventional disease-modifying antirheumatic drugs (DMARDs) play a dominant role in the treatment of rheumatoid arthritis, but they have no proven efficacy for the axial manifestations of AS. Figure 6.6 summarizes three studies with sulfasalazine, leflunomide, and methotrexate in AS, clearly showing that there is no improvement in the disease activity in these patients [14–17]. DMARDs have a limited efficacy for the peripheral manifestations in AS; the best data are available for sulfasalazine given at a dose of 2–3 g/day orally [18].

Anti-tumor necrosis factor-alpha-blocking agents in ankylosing spondylitis

It can be estimated that about 20% of patients with AS are still active despite optimal treatment with NSAIDs. This means that the demonstration of good or very good efficacy of TNF blockers in the treatment of patients with active AS can be regarded as a breakthrough in the therapy of these

Conventional disease-modifying antirheumatic drugs are not effective for the treatment of ankylosing spondylitis

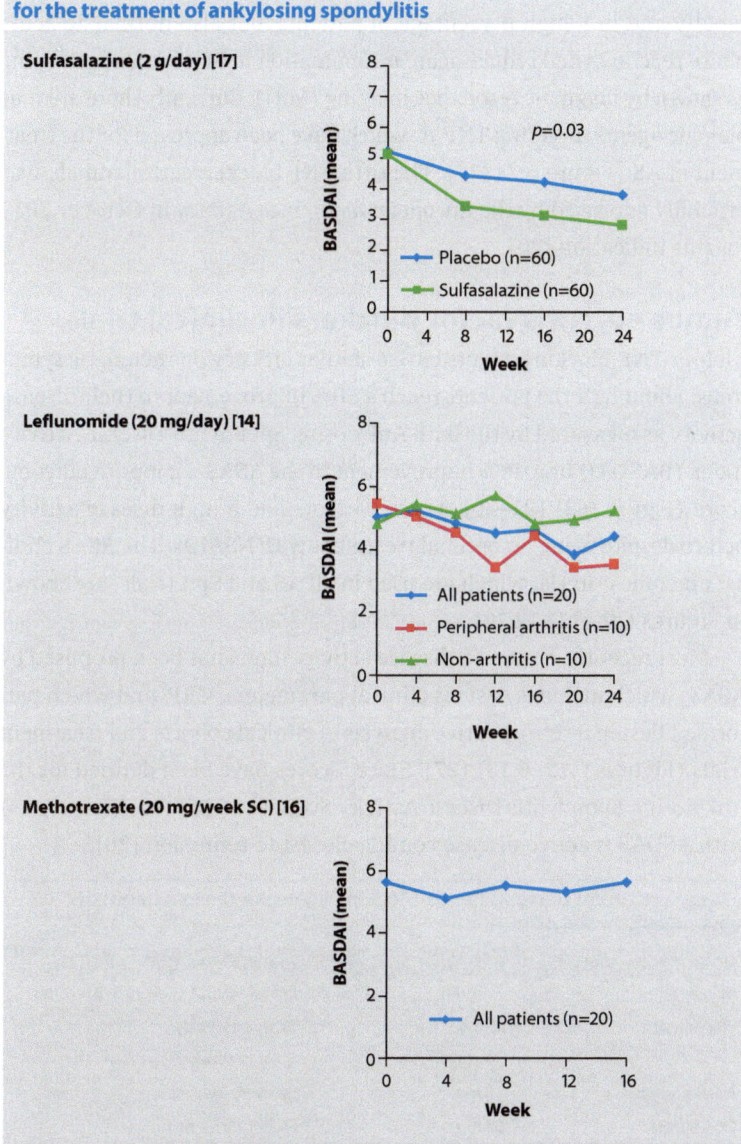

Figure 6.6 Conventional disease-modifying antirheumatic drugs are not effective for the treatment of ankylosing spondylitis. BASDAI, Bath Ankylosing Spondylitis Disease Activity Index; SC, subcutaneous. Adapted from Haibel et al [14], Haibel et al [16], Braun J et al [17].

patients with AS. These drugs not only improve signs and symptoms rapidly and in a high percentage of patients, but also normalize acute phase reactants and reduce acute inflammation in SI joints and the spine as shown by magnetic resonance imaging (MRI). Currently there are four biologic agents targeting TNF-α, which have been approved for the treatment of AS (Figure 6.7) [19]. The fifth TNF blocker, certolizumab, was officially approved by the European Medicines Agency in October 2013 for this indication [20].

Tumor necrosis factor blockers in clinical trials

All four TNF-blocking agents have a similar efficacy on rheumatic symptoms: about half the patients reach a 50% improvement in their disease activity as measured by the Bath Ankylosing Spondylitis Disease Activity Index (BASDAI) or a 40% improvement in the ASAS composite outcome score (Figure 6.8) [21–26]. These patients had a high disease activity before despite being on optimal treatment with NSAIDs. The ASAS clinical outcome criteria, which are used in all AS and SpA trials, are shown in Figures 6.9–6.11 [2,19].

Most recently, a new AS disease activity index has been proposed by ASAS, which includes besides clinical parameters, CRP, and which performed best in a retrospective analysis of clinical cohorts and treatment trials (Figures 6.12, 6.13) [27]. Status scores have been defined for the Ankylosing Spondylitis Disease Activity Score (ASDAS) (see Figure 6.14) with ASDAS inactive disease coming closest to remission [28].

Dosage of tumor necrosis factor-blocking agents in the treatment of ankylosing spondylitis		
Drug	**AS**	**Application**
Infliximab	5 mg/kg	IV at week 0, 2, 6, every 6–8 weeks
Etanercept	25 mg	SC twice weekly
	50 mg	SC once weekly
Adalimumab	40 mg	SC every 2 weeks
Golimumab	50 mg	SC once a month
Certolizumab	200 mg or	SC every 2 weeks or
	400mg	SC every 4 weeks

Figure 6.7 Dosage of tumor necrosis factor-blocking agents in the treatment of ankylosing spondylitis. AS, ankylosing spondylitis; IV, intravenous; SC, subcutaneous.

Impressive reduction of inflammatory lesions either in the SI joints or in the spine have been demonstrated for all four TNF blockers (Figures 6.15–6.18) [29–31].

Interestingly, there is still a further decrease of inflammation if patients are treated over 2 years, although in a small proportion of patients inflammation, as seen by MRI, is not suppressed completely [32]. AS and related SpA seem to be the disease for which TNF blockers are most effective, probably more effective than in rheumatoid arthritis [33]. Long-term follow-up of patients with AS treated with TNF blockers (Figures 6.19 and 6.20) has to date been published for up to 8 years, showing good long-term efficacy if treatment is continued [23,24,34–38]. A drop-out rate of about 10% per year can be expected for patients on long-term treatment, for various reasons, such as side effects, loss of efficacy, or lack of compliance. However, when treatment was stopped, nearly all these patients with long-standing active disease showed a flare-up. It still has to be seen whether this is the case when patients are treated earlier.

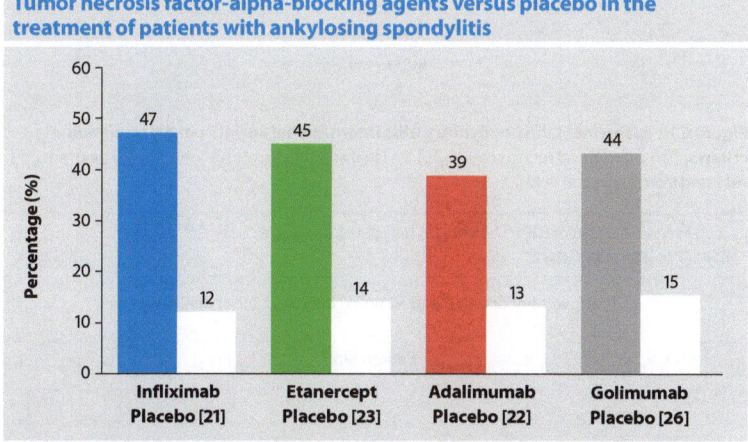

Figure 6.8 Tumor necrosis factor-alpha-blocking agents versus placebo in the treatment of patients with ankylosing spondylitis. Different studies, no head-to-head comparison. Response to treatment at 24 weeks was defined using Assessment in SpondyloArthritis international Society response criteria 40 (ie, 40% improvement from baseline). Adapted from van der Heijde et al [21], van der Heijde et al [22], Davis et al [23], Inman et al [26]. Reproduced with permission from © ASAS [www.asas-group.org]. All Rights Reserved.

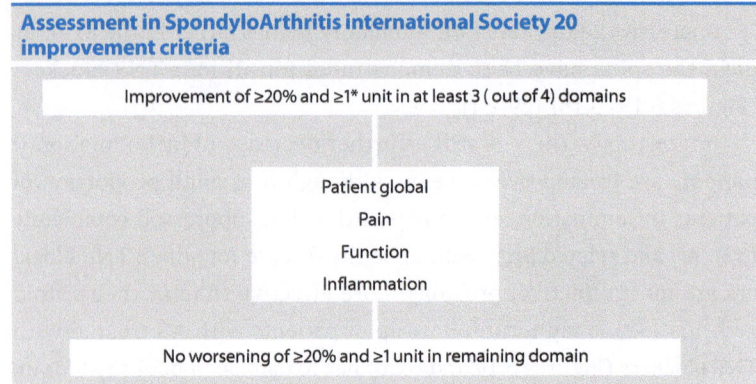

Figure 6.9 Assessment in SpondyloArthritis international Society 20 improvement criteria. *On a numerical rating scale (0–10). A visual analogue scale (0–100) can also be used. Adapted from Anderson et al [2].

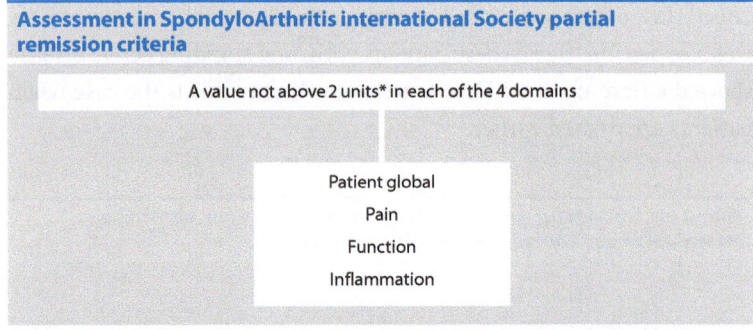

Figure 6.10 Assessment in SpondyloArthritis international Society partial remission criteria. *On a numerical rating scale (0–10). A visual analogue scale (0–100) can also be used. Adapted from Anderson et al [2].

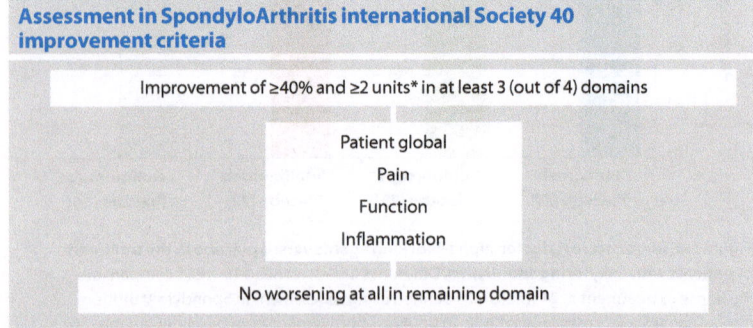

Figure 6.11 Assessment in SpondyloArthritis international Society 40 improvement criteria. *On a numerical rating scale (0–10). A visual analogue scale (0–100) can also be used. Reproduced with permission from Brandt et al [19].

Ankylosing spondylitis disease score I

Parameters used for the calculation of the AS disease activity score

1. Total back pain (BASDAI question 2)

2. Patient global (on a scale 0–10)

3. Peripheral pain/swelling (BASDAI question 3)

4. Duration of morning stiffness (BASDAI question 6)

5. C-reactive protein in mg/l (or erythrocyte sedimentation rate)

Figure 6.12 Ankylosing spondylitis disease score I. AS, ankylosing spondylitis; BASDAI, Bath Ankylosing Spondylitis Disease Activity Index. Reproduced with permission from © BMJ Publishing Group Ltd. 2013, van der Heijde et al [27]. All Rights Reserved.

Ankylosing spondylitis disease activity score II calculation

$ASDAS_{CRP}$

$0.121 \times$ total back pain $+ 0.110 \times$ patient global $+ 0.073 \times$ peripheral pain/swelling $+ 0.058 \times$ duration of morning stiffness $+ 0.579 \times Ln(CRP+1)$

$ASDAS_{ESR}$

$0.113 \times$ patient global $+ 0.293 \times \sqrt{ESR} + 0.086 \times$ peripheral pain/swelling $+ 0.069 \times$ duration of morning stiffness $+ 0.079 \times$ total back pain

The $ASDAS_{CRP}$ is the preferred ASDAS but the $ASDAS_{ESR}$ can be used in case CRP is not available. CRP in mg/l; all patient assessments are on a 10 cm scale.

Figure 6.13 Ankylosing spondylitis disease activity score II calculation.
ASDAS, ankylosing spondylitis disease activity score; CRP, C-reactive protein; ESR, erythrocyte sedimentation rate. Reproduced with permission from © BMJ Publishing Group Ltd. 2013, van der Heijde et al [27]. All Rights Reserved.

Ankylosing Spondylitis Disease Activity Score cut-offs for status score

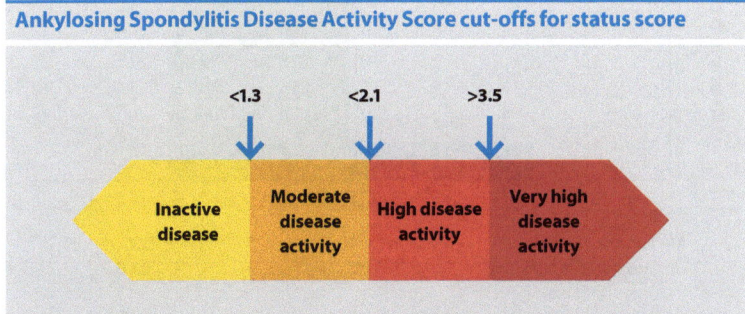

Figure 6.14 Ankylosing Spondylitis Disease Activity Score cut-offs for status score.
Reproduced with permission from © BMJ Publishing Group Ltd. 2013, Machado et al [28]. All Rights Reserved.

Effects of infliximab therapy on ankylosing spondylitis

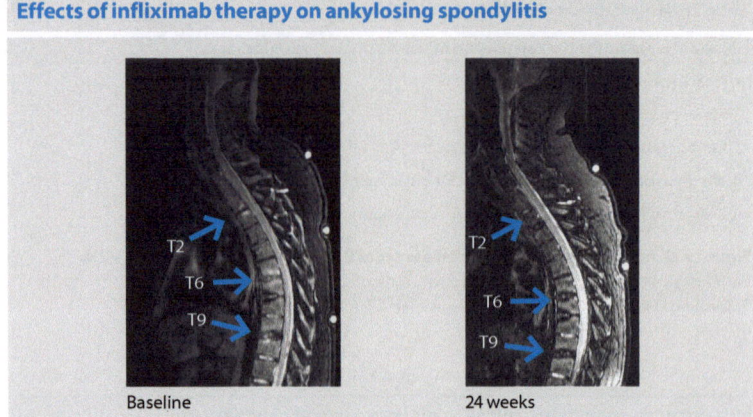

Baseline   24 weeks

Figure 6.15 Effects of infliximab therapy on ankylosing spondylitis. MRI images of the thoracic vertebrae of a patient with ankylosing spondylitis at baseline and after 24 weeks of infliximab therapy. Reproduced with permission from © John Wiley and Sons 2013, Braun et al [29]. All Rights Reserved.

Ankylosing Spondylitis Study for the Evaluation of Recombinant infliximab Therapy: Improvement from baseline in MRI activity score (short tau inversion recovery) at week 24

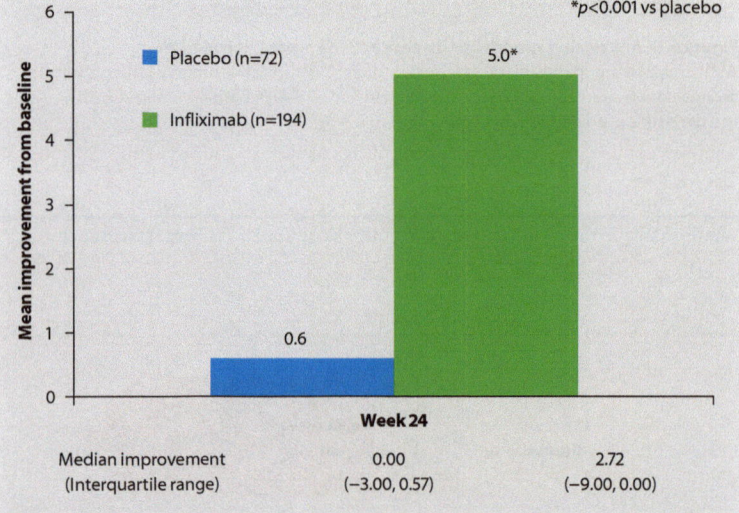

Figure 6.16 Ankylosing Spondylitis Study for the Evaluation of Recombinant infliximab Therapy: Improvement from baseline in MRI activity score (short tau inversion recovery) at week 24. Adapted from Braun et al [29].

Sacroiliac joints before and after etanercept treatment

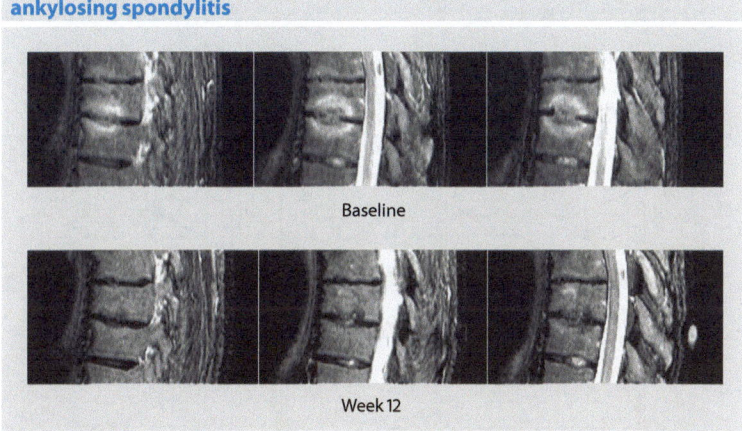

Before — After 6 weeks — After 24 weeks

Figure 6.17 Sacroiliac joints before and after etanercept treatment. Reproduced with permission from © BMJ Publishing Group Ltd. 2013, Rudwaleit et al [30]. All Rights Reserved.

Adalimumab reduces inflammation in the spine of patient with ankylosing spondylitis

Baseline

Week 12

Figure 6.18 Adalimumab reduces inflammation in the spine of patient with ankylosing spondylitis. Reproduced with permission from © John Wiley and Sons 2013, Lambert et al [31]. All Rights Reserved.

Adverse events of tumor necrosis factor blockers

The adverse events in patients with AS treated with TNF blockers do not differ from those seen in other diseases, such as rheumatoid arthritis and Crohn's disease. However, patients with AS are normally younger and have been less frequently treated with glucocorticoids or immunosuppressive drugs compared with the other two diseases. Thus, the number and the severity of side effects can be expected to be at least no higher than for other chronic inflammatory diseases, but possibly even lower.

Efficacy of tumor necrosis factor-antagonists in patients with ankylosing spondylitis

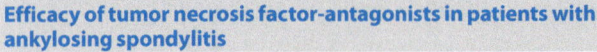

Infliximab (ASSERT) [34]

Responders (%) — Weeks

n= 201 199 166

Etanercept [23]

Responders (%) — Weeks

n= 138 128 95

Adalimumab (ATLAS) [35]

Responders (%) — Weeks

n= 311 296 261

Golimumab (GO-RAISE) [37]

Responders (%) — Weeks

n=number of patients on therapy

◆ ASAS 20   ■ ASAS 40   ■ ASAS partial remission

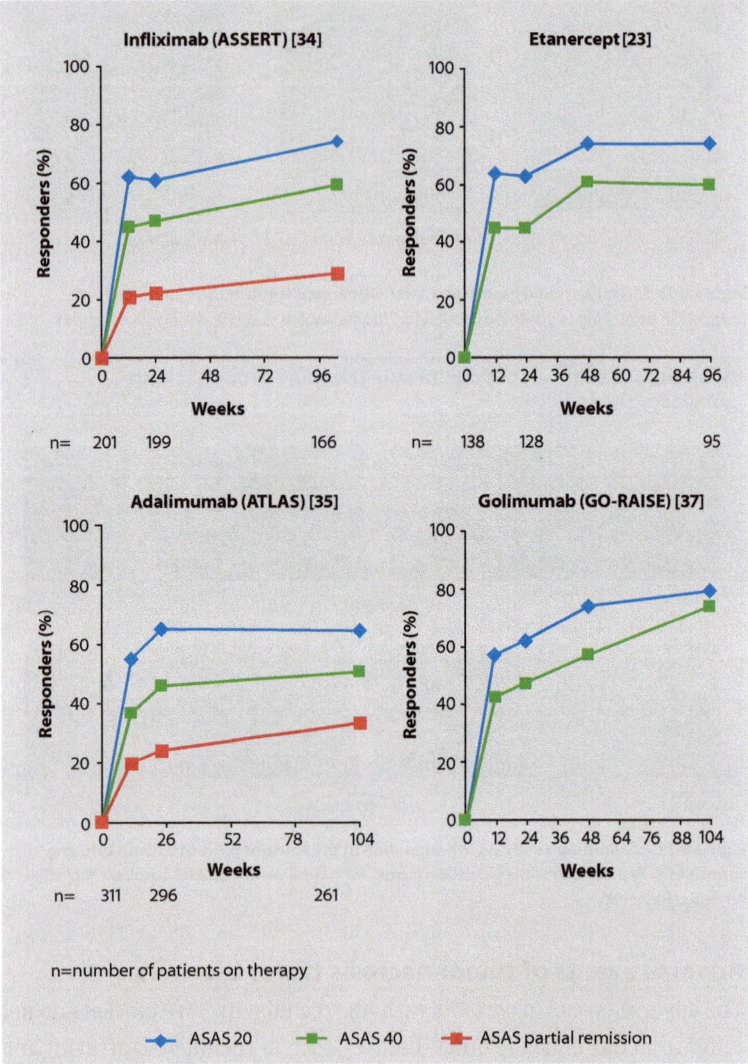

Figure 6.19 Efficacy of tumor necrosis factor-antagonists in patients with ankylosing spondylitis. Golimumab group shown here received initial 50 mg every 4 weeks. ASAS, Assessment in SpondyloArthritis international Society. Reproduced with permission from © BMJ Publishing Group Ltd. 2013, from Davis et al [23], All Rights Reserved; Adapted from Braun et al [34]; Adapted from van der Heijde et al [35]; Reproduced with permission from © BMJ Publishing Group Ltd. 2013, Braun et al [37], All Rights Reserved. Reproduced with permission from © ASAS [www.asas-group.org]. All Rights Reserved.

Long-term clinical efficacy of tumor necrosis factor blocker in patients with ankylosing spondylitis, results over 8 years

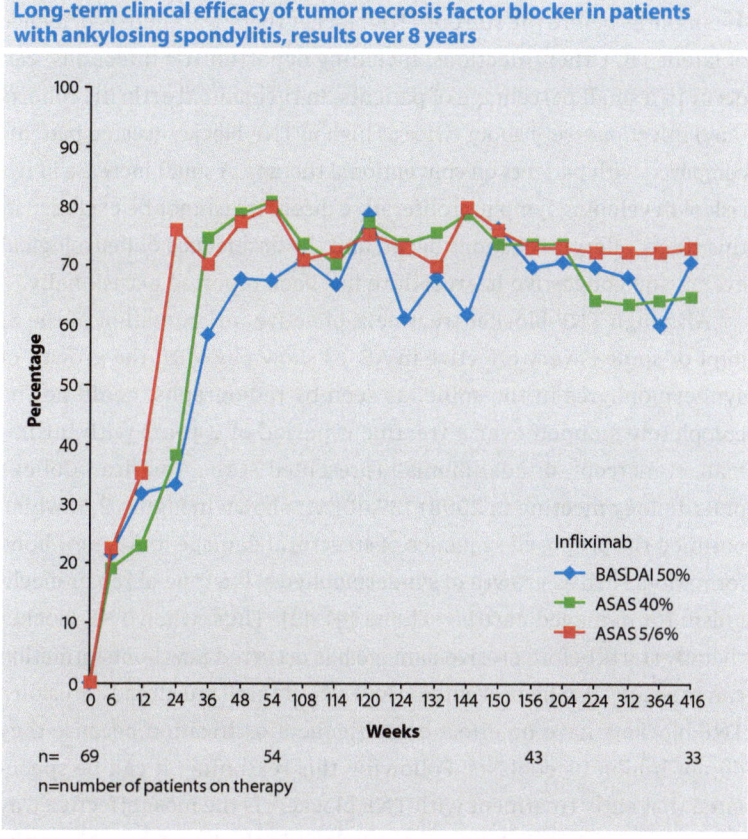

Figure 6.20 Long-term clinical efficacy of tumor necrosis factor blocker in patients with ankylosing spondylitis, results over 8 years. ASAS, Assessment in SpondyloArthritis international Society; BASDAI, Bath Ankylosing Spondylitis Disease Activity Index. Adapted from Braun J et al [24], Baraliakos X et al [36], Braun et al [38].

Comparative data on this are not available at this time, but application and implementation of the usual precautions and contraindications for biologic therapy should be followed, especially screening for latent tuberculosis (TB) before anti-TNF therapy is initiated.

According to most national guidelines a patient's history should be taken, a radiograph of the chest performed, and immune response to TB tested either by tuberculin skin test and/or an in vitro T-cell assay for TB-specific antigens. Normally, patients are treated with 300 mg isoniazide for 9 months or alternatively with 600 mg rifampicin for

4–6 months before the start of TNF-blocker therapy if there is evidence of latent TB. Other infections, including opportunistic infections, can occur in a small percentage of patients. In rheumatoid arthritis cohorts (any) infections were about twice as high in TNF-blocker-treated patients compared with patients on conventional therapy. A small increase in the risk of developing lymphoproliferative disorders cannot be excluded at this stage, allergic reactions occur, and the occurrence of neurological events and congestive heart failure has been reported occasionally.

Although TNF-blocker treatment of active inflammation of the SI joint or spine is very effective in AS, as shown by MRI, the growth of syndesmophytes in the spine, as seen by radiographs, could not be completely stopped over a treatment period of 2 years with infliximab, etanercept, or adalimumab (presented at the American College of Radiology meeting in 2008) [39,40]. As shown in Figure 2.8, which outlined the proposed sequence of structural damage in AS, new bone formation, such as growth of syndesmophytes, is a type of repair mechanism for damaged cartilage/bone [41,42]. Thus, when TNF-blocker therapy starts before erosive damage has occurred new bone formation can probably also be prevented. However, if there are already erosions, TNF blockers have no effect on subsequent ossification because they do not inhibit osteoblasts. Following this reasoning, it can be speculated that early treatment with TNF blockers is the most effective way to prevent syndesmophytes and ankylosis in the long term. Along the same line, a window of opportunity for early TNF-blocker treatment has recently been proposed [43]. Two recent studies do also suggest that an inhibitory effect on new bone formation by TNF blockers might become only visible after several years (>4 years) of treatment [44,45]. However, this still has to be further proven by additional studies. Furthermore, the observed small growth of syndesmophytes is probably not clinically meaningful because it has been shown that in the same patients function and spinal mobility improved over 2 years of treatment [34,46].

In contrast to the treatment of rheumatoid arthritis, there is no evidence that combination of a TNF blocker with a conventional DMARD is superior compared with treatment of AS with a TNF blocker alone.

Most of the patients in the studies were indeed treated with TNF-blocker monotherapy. Two recent studies comparing infliximab alone versus infliximab plus methotrexate showed clearly that there was no significant difference between the two groups regarding efficacy and side effects [47,48].

Extrarheumatic manifestations or comorbidities, such as uveitis, psoriasis, or inflammatory bowel disease (IBD), are present or have occurred in the past in 40–50% of patients with AS [49]. Thus, it is also interesting whether the three TNF blockers differ in their efficacy with regard to these manifestations. Both monoclonal antibodies have been shown to be effective for the treatment of Crohn's disease, and infliximab for ulcerative colitis, whereas etanercept does not work in IBD. When it was investigated whether TNF blockers reduce flares or a new onset of IBD in patients with AS treated for their rheumatic manifestations, infliximab was clearly superior to etanercept whereas the number of patients treated with adalimumab was too small in this meta-analysis to allow any further conclusions [50]. In another meta-analysis of trials from patients with AS treated with TNF blockers both infliximab and etanercept reduced flares of uveitis, but infliximab was slightly more effective [51]. Based on data from a small retrospective study and from one large but uncontrolled observational study, adalimumab seems also to reduce flares of uveitis, from 15 flares per 100 patient-years before treatment to 7.4 in one of the studies [52]. All three TNF blockers are effective for psoriasis, although infliximab shows the best efficacy on the skin in the doses normally used for the treatment of AS.

Failure of tumor necrosis factor-blocker treatment and switching to another agent

Antidrug antibodies can develop, especially against the monoclonal antibodies. Recently a structured approach in case of inefficacy of TNF-blocker treatment has been proposed [53]. Dependent on antidrug antibody levels and TNF-blocker serum levels either a dose increase or a switch to another TNF blocker is suggested. However, the real clinical relevance of antidrug antibodies and its clinical application has still to be better defined.

An ASAS 40 response rate can be expected in 38% of patients (compared to 59% in case of no prior TNF-blocker exposure) if treatment is switched from one TNF blocker to another in one investigation. Patients respond better if response is lost over time compared with patients who show no response at the start of treatment [54]. In another report a decrease of the BASDAI by two points was still observed in patients who switched to a second and third TNF blocker in comparison to a decrease of three BASDAI points in patients on their first TNF blocker [55].

Several other biologics have been investigated for the treatment of AS but most of them have failed so far. The interleukin (IL)-1 receptor antagonist anakinra [14] and the T-cell modulating drug abatacept [56] could not show any effect in two prospective open-label trials over 6 months in patients with active AS. Furthermore, the monoclonal antibody tocilizumab, directed against the IL-6 receptor, did not show any effect at all in TNF-naïve patients in a placebo-controlled double blind study [57]. In another small open label trial treatment the B-cell antagonist rituximab showed a higher than expected effect in TNF-naïve patients but not in TNF-failure patients, a finding which has to be further investigated in a placebo-controlled study. Interestingly, the IL-17 antagonist secukinumab was superior to placebo in active AS [58]. However, this result was obtained in a small study and has to be confirmed in currently ongoing larger trials. Thus, there are no alternative biologics available at the moment in patients who fail TNF-blocker therapy, with IL-17 and probably also IL-23 currently the most promising treatment targets.

The use of tumor necrosis factor blockers in nonradiographic axial spondyloarthritis

With the good response of the patients with AS to TNF blockers the question came up whether improvement can even be increased if patients were treated earlier and whether patients in their nr-axSpA stage respond similarly well or even better. There are now three TNF-blocker trials in patients with nr-axSpA and several other studies treating the whole axSpA group with TNF inhibitors, including nr-axSpA and AS. If nr-axSpA patients were treated with adalimumab for 12 weeks an ASAS 40 response was achieved in 54% of patients versus 12% in the placebo group, an effect that was maintained over 1 year of treatment for the whole group after the placebo patients were also switched to adalimumab (see Figure 6.21) [59]. In the subgroup of patients with a disease duration of less than 3 years such a major response was achieved in 80% of patients. This result was recently confirmed in a larger placebo-controlled trial with adalimumab in nr-axSpA over 12 weeks with an open label extension phase [60]. Interestingly, patients with symptom duration less than 5 years, elevated CRP or – to a lesser extent – active inflammation on MRI responded better (see Figure 6.22) [60]. Based on these trials adalimumab was the first TNF blocker which has been approved in the European Commission for the treatment of adults with severe axSpA without radiographic evidence of AS but with objective signs of inflammation by elevated CRP and/or MRI, who have had an inadequate response to or are intolerant to NSAIDs. A recent study with etanercept in active patients with nr-axSpA reported also a clear superiority of the

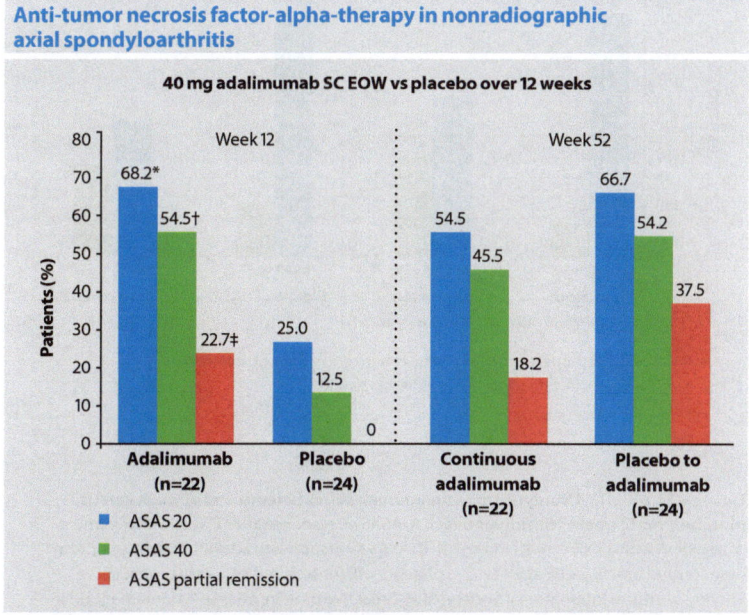

Figure 6.21 Anti-tumor necrosis factor-alpha-therapy in nonradiographic axial spondyloarthritis. *p=0.007; †p=0.004; ‡p=0.019. ASAS, Assessment in SpondyloArthritis international Society; EOW, end of week; SC, subcutaneous. Reproduced with permission from © John Wiley and Sons 2013, Haibel H et al [59]. All Rights Reserved.

ABILITY-I Study: 40 mg adalimumab subcutaneous end of week versus placebo over 12 weeks (continues over)

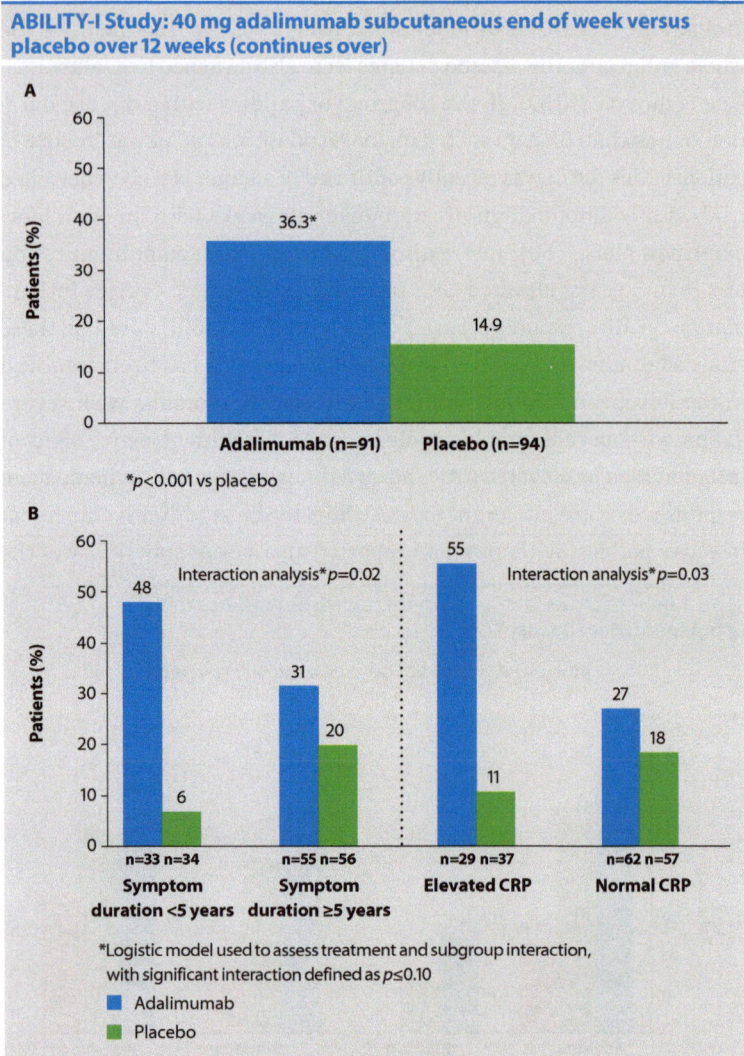

Figure 6.22 ABILITY-I Study: 40 mg adalimumab subcutaneous end of week versus placebo over 12 weeks (continues over). A, ASAS 40 response after 12 weeks of treatment of nr-axSpA with a TNF-α-blocking agent; B, ASAS 40 response to adalimumab by symptom duration and baseline CRP at week 12 in patients with nr-axSpA. ASAS, Assessment in SpondyloArthritis international Society; CRP, C-reactive protein; nr-axSpA, nonradiographic axial spondyloarthritis. Reproduced with permission from © BMJ Publishing Group Ltd. 2013, Sieper J et al [60]. All Rights Reserved.

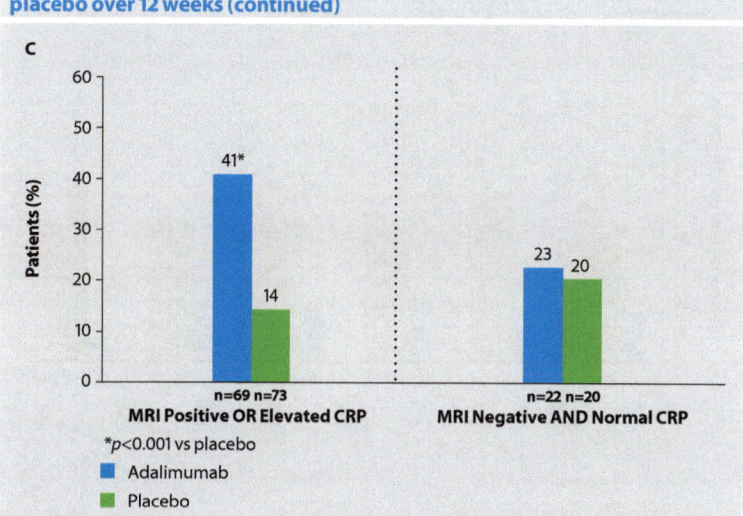

ABILITY-I Study: 40 mg adalimumab subcutaneous end of week versus placebo over 12 weeks (continued)

Figure 6.22 ABILITY-I Study: 40 mg adalimumab subcutaneous end of week versus placebo over 12 weeks (continued). C, ASAS 40 response to adalimumab by baseline MRI and CRP at week 12 in patients with nr-axSpA. ASAS, Assessment in SpondyloArthritis international Society; CRP, C-reactive protein; nr-axSpA, nonradiographic axial spondyloarthritis. Reproduced with permission from © BMJ Publishing Group Ltd. 2013, Sieper J et al [60]. All Rights Reserved.

TNF blocker compared to placebo [61]. Most recently also the TNF-blocker certolizumab was approved in the EC for this indication [20] (see Figure 6.23). Another trial with the TNF blocker golimumab for this indication is still ongoing.

Three other studies with early axSpA, including both patients with radiographic (AS) and nr-axSpA, with symptom duration of less than 3 or 5 years, resulted in clinical remission rates of 50% or more when treated with infliximab (see Figure 6.24) [5,62] or etanercept [63]. The treatment response was identical in the etanercept study when patients with AS and nr-axSpA were compared, clearly indicating that the response to TNF-blocker therapy is about the same for the two groups if the level of objective inflammation, such as elevated CRP and MRI-inflammation, is the same [64]. Finally, a placebo-controlled double blind study was performed in patients with active axSpA with the TNF blocker certolizumab, about half of the patients with radiographic sacroiliitis (AS) and the other half with nr-axSpA. Symptom duration was not limited in

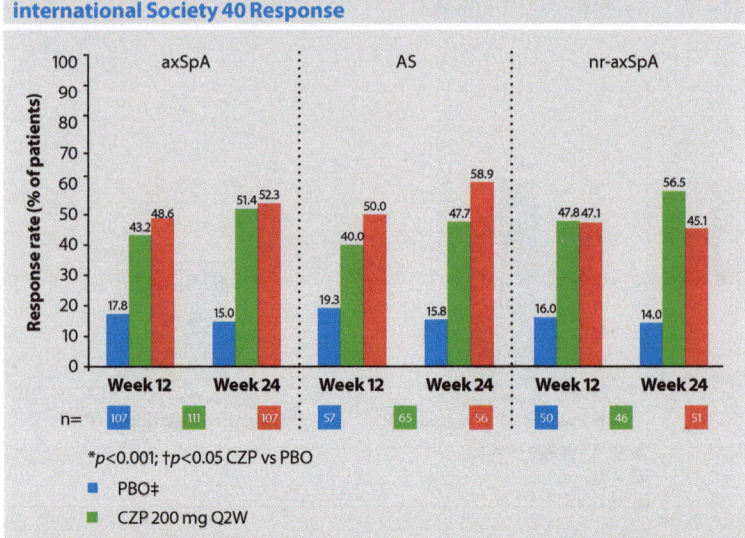

Figure 6.23 Certolizumab in axial spondyloarthritis Assessment in SpondyloArthritis international Society 40 Response. axSpA, axial spondyloarthritis; AS, ankylosing spondylitis; CZP, certolizumab; nr-axSpA, nonradiographic axial spondyloarthritis; PBO, placebo. Reproduced with permission from © BMJ Publishing Group Ltd. 2013, Landewe et al [20]. All Rights Reserved.

this study; however, all patients had to have either an elevated CRP or active inflammation of the SI joint on MRI. The response rate and the difference to the placebo group were comparable with the other axSpA and nr-axSpA trials. But most interestingly, the treatment effect was the same in AS and nr-axSpA subgroups [20].

When patients with nr-axSpA or axSpA with a short symptom duration being in remission or having achieved a good clinical response were taken off etanercept [65] or adalimumab [66] 69% and 83%, respectively, relapsed, with again showing a good response when TNF-blocker therapy was restarted. When infliximab was given in patients with active axSpA at first-line therapy in combination with an NSAIDs in patients who were not yet NSAIDs failures for 24 weeks treatment was stopped after 6 months. Patients who reached remission were randomized to be not treated at all or with naproxen 1000 mg/day for another 6 months. The relapse was similar with 40% and 47.5% respectively, between these

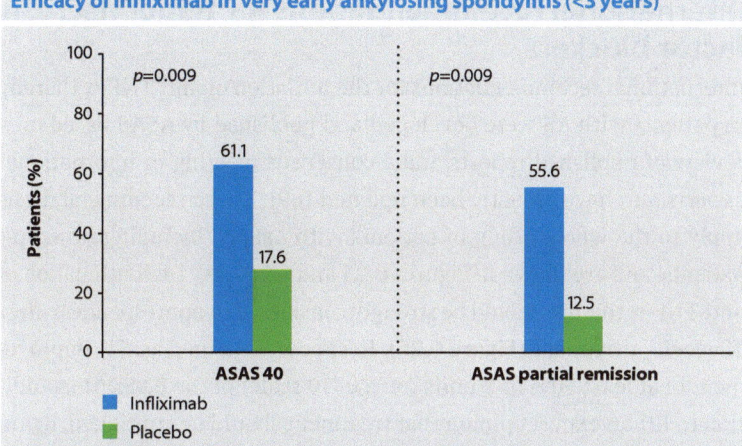

Figure 6.24 Efficacy of infliximab in very early ankylosing spondylitis (<3 years). Significant improvements in clinical end points compared with placebo at 16 weeks. Diagnostic criteria: inflammatory back pain, HLA-B27 positive, and bone edema on MRI. Mean symptom duration was 15.3 months. ASAS, Assessment in SpondyloArthritis international Society; HLA, human leukocyte antigen. Adapted from Barkham et al [62].

two groups. But interestingly, 87.1% and 93.8% of patients, respectively, remained in a status of low clinical disease activity defined as a BASDAI always <3 [67]. Thus, although the majority of patients with nr-axSpA or early axSpA relapse when TNF-blocker therapy is withdrawn, there seems to be a trend to higher drug-free remission rates in patients treated earlier.

Tumor necrosis factor blockers in the treatment of juvenile spondyloarthritis

The first symptoms of AS occur in 15–20% of cases before the age of 20 years and juvenile and adult spondyloarthritis should be seen as one disease with a continuum. While the juvenile forms normally present first with a predominance of peripheral manifestations (enthesitis and peripheral arthritis), many of the juvenile patients later develop the full picture of typical AS. Both infliximab and etanercept have shown good efficacy in patients with juvenile SpA or enthesitis-related arthritis in smaller studies. A recent placebo-controlled small trial could also show a good efficacy for adalimumab in patients with juvenile onset AS [68].

International recommendations for tumor necrosis factor blockers

International recommendations for the initiation of anti-TNF-α therapy in patients with AS were developed and published by ASAS based on a review of published reports and a consensus meeting of international experts and have recently been updated [69]. These recommendations apply to the whole group of patients with axSpA, including nr-axSpA patients, and are shown in Figures 6.25 and 6.26 [69]. Discontinuation of anti-TNF-α therapy should be strongly considered in nonresponders after 12 weeks' treatment (Figure 6.26). Response is defined as: (1) improvement of at least 50% or 2 units (on a 0–10 scale) of the BASDAI in addition to (2) an expert opinion that treatment should be continued, again not just relying on patients' subjective symptoms.

Similar recommendations or guidelines have been published by national societies, such as the British Society for Rheumatology (Figure 6.27) the Canadian Rheumatology Association (Figure 6.28), and the Spondylitis Association of America (Figure 6.29), following the reasoning of the ASAS recommendations, only with slight modifications [70–72]. However, these recommendations are still restricted to AS.

Prediction of a good response to tumor necrosis factor-blocker treatment

When an analysis was made of which parameters predict a response to TNF blockers best, short disease duration and/or young age were the best predictors, indicating that patients with long-lasting disease also have causes other than inflammation contributing to the clinical symptoms [59,73]. An elevated CRP and active inflammation, as shown by MRI, were also predictive, although not as good as short disease duration and young age [74]. The high response rates in three studies in patients with axSpA with a symptom duration of less than 3–5 years and the presence of active bony inflammation on MRI on inclusion also suggest that short symptom duration (and/or young age) and the presence of objective signs of inflammation, such as a positive MRI, are currently the best predictors of a response to TNF-blockers.

Assessment in SpondyloArthritis international Society recommendations for the use of anti-tumor necrosis factor-agents in patients with axial spondyloarthritis

Diagnosis: fulfillment of the modified New York criteria for AS or the ASAS criteria for axSpA

Predominant axial manifestations →

Failure of standard treatment:
- at least 2 NSAIDs over 4 weeks (in total)
- one local steroid injection if appropriate ← Predominant peripheral manifestations
- normally a therapeutic trial of a DMARD, preferably sulfasalazine (not mandatory) ←

High disease activity: BASDAI ≥4

plus

Positive expert opinion based on parameters such as:
- Positive CRP/ESR
- Positive MRI
- Radiological progression
- Clinical examination

Figure 6.25 Assessment in SpondyloArthritis international Society recommendations for the use of anti-tumor necrosis factor-agents in patients with axial spondyloarthritis. AS, ankylosing spondylitis; ASAS, Assessment in SpondyloArthritis international Society; axSpA, axial spondyloarthritis; BASDAI, Bath Ankylosing Spondylitis Disease Activity Index; CRP, C-reactive protein; DMARD, disease-modifying antirheumatic drug; ESR, erythrocyte sedimentation rate; NSAID, nonsteroidal anti-inflammatory drug. Adapted from van der Heijde et al [69].

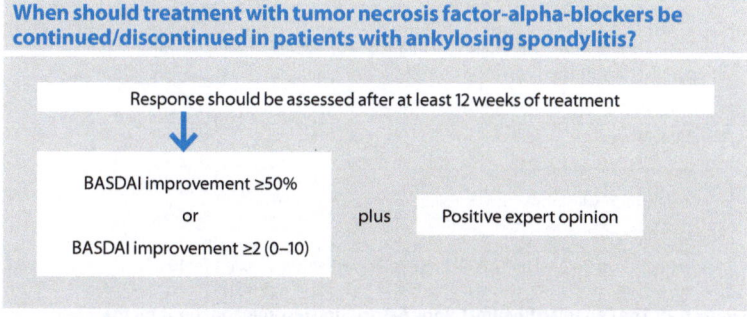

When should treatment with tumor necrosis factor-alpha-blockers be continued/discontinued in patients with ankylosing spondylitis?

Response should be assessed after at least 12 weeks of treatment ↓

BASDAI improvement ≥50%

or

BASDAI improvement ≥2 (0–10)

plus Positive expert opinion

Figure 6.26 When should treatment with tumor necrosis factor-alpha-blockers be continued/discontinued in patients with ankylosing spondylitis? BASDAI, Bath Ankylosing Spondylitis Disease Activity Index. Adapted from van der Heije et al [69].

British Society for Rheumatology guidelines for prescribing tumor necrosis factor blockers in the treatment of ankylosing spondylitis

- Diagnosis
  - Modified New York criteria
- Disease activity
  - BASDAI at least 4 (scale 0–10)
  - And spinal pain (VAS 0–10) at least 4 cm
  - Both on two occasions at least 4 weeks apart without any change of treatment
- Previous treatment
  - Failure of conventional treatment with two or more NSAIDs, each taken sequentially at maximum tolerated/recommended dosage for 4 weeks
- Criteria for withdrawl
  - Development of severe side effects
  - Inefficacy, as indicated by failure of the BASDAI to improve by 50% or to fall at least 2 units and/or for the spinal pain VAS to reduce by at least 2 units after 3 months

Figure 6.27 British Society for Rheumatology guidelines for prescribing tumor necrosis factor blockers in the treatment of ankylosing spondylitis. BASDAI, Bath Ankylosing Spondylitis Disease Activity Index; NSAID, nonsteroidal anti-inflammatory drug; VAS, visual analogue scale. Adapted from Keat et al [70].

The Canadian Rheumatology Association recommendations for the treatment of ankylosing spondylitis with tumor necrosis factor blockers

- Anti-TNF treatment should be given under supervision of a rheumatologist
- Failure of conventional treatment
  - At least 3 NSAIDs, each administered over a minimum 2-week period at accepted maximum dosage if tolerated
  - There is no evidence to support the obligatory use of DMARDs before or together with TNF blockers
  - Sulfasalazine and/or methotrexate might be considered in patients with peripheral arthritis
- Disease activity (at least two of the following)
  - BASDAI >4
  - Elevated CRP and/or ESR
  - Inflammatory lesions in the sacroiliac joint and/or spine on MRI
- Responder criteria
  - Reduction of BASDAI by 2 (0–10) or a relative reduction of 50% after 16 weeks

Figure 6.28 The Canadian Rheumatology Association recommendations for the treatment of ankylosing spondylitis with tumor necrosis factor blockers. BASDAI, Bath Ankylosing Spondylitis Disease Activity Index; CRP, C-reactive protein; DMARD, disease-modifying antirheumatic drug; ESR, erythrocyte sedimentation rate; NSAID, nonsteroidal anti-inflammatory drug; TNF, tumor necrosis factor. Adapted from Maksymowych et al [71].

The Spondylitis Association of America guidelines for the use of anti-tumor necrosis factor therapy in patients with ankylosing spondylitis

- Diagnosis: modified New York criteria
- Disease activity
  - BASDAI ≥4 (scale 0–10)
  - Physician global assessment of ≥2 on a Likert scale: 0=none, 1=mild, 2=moderate, 3=severe, 4=very severe
- Failure of previous treatment
  - Failure by lack of response or intolerability to ≥2 NSAIDs for at least 3 months for all three presentations: axial, peripheral arthritis, enthesitis
  - Patients with peripheral arthritis must have had a lack of response to >1 DMARD (sulfasalazine preferred). Not required for axial disease or enthesitis (steroid injection not required)
- Dosing
  - Etanercept 2x25 mg sq twice a week (note from the authors: a dosing of 50 mg sq once a week was not yet available when these recommendations were published)
  - Infliximab 5 mg /kg IV every 6–8 weeks
  - Adalimumab (note from the authors: this drug was not yet approved when these recommendations were published; normal dosing: 40 mg sq every 2 weeks)
- Responder criteria
  - Improvement of BASDAI by at least 2 units and Physician's Global >1
- Time of evaluation
  - 6–8 weeks
- Tuberculosis precautions
  - Tuberculosis screening and treatment as indicated by the American Thoracic Association

Figure 6.29 The Spondylitis Association of America guidelines for the use of anti-tumor necrosis factor therapy in patients with ankylosing spondylitis. BASDAI, Bath Ankylosing Spondylitis Disease Activity Index; DMARD, disease-modifying antirheumatic drugs; IV, intravenous; NSAID, nonsteroidal anti-inflammatory drug. Adapted from Spondylitis Association of America [72].

Which instruments should be used for clinical record keeping?

The BASDAI is a questionnaire filled in by the patient – covering fatigue, back pain, peripheral joint pain, pain of entheses, and morning stiffness – and is normally used for the assessment of disease activity (Figure 6.30) [75]. It does not help to differentiate AS from other causes of back pain but gives a good estimate of the level of disease activity in a patient with AS, if symptoms are caused by inflammation. In addition to the BASDAI, ASAS has proposed a core set for clinical record keeping, which is shown in Figure 6.31 [76]. The functional index BASFI (Bath Ankylosing

Bath Ankylosing Spondylitis Disease Activity Index

NRS BASDI

Please tick the box which represents your answer.

All questions refer to **last week** (ie, ☒)

1. How would you describe the overall level of fatigue/tiredness you have experienced?

| 0 | 1 | 2 | 3 | 4 | ☒ | 6 | 7 | 8 | 9 | 10 |

none   very severe

Fatigue

2. How would you describe the overall level of AS **neck, back, or hip** pain you have had?

| 0 | 1 | 2 | 3 | 4 | 5 | 6 | ☒ | 8 | 9 | 10 |

none   very severe

Spinal pain

3. How would you describe the overall level of pain/swelling in joints **other than** neck, back, or hips you have had?

| 0 | ☒ | 2 | 3 | 4 | 5 | 6 | 7 | 8 | 9 | 10 |

none   very severe

Peripheral arthritis

4. How would you describe the overall level of discomfort you have had from any areas tender to touch or pressure?

| 0 | 1 | ☒ | 3 | 4 | 5 | 6 | 7 | 8 | 9 | 10 |

none   very severe

Enthestis

5. How would you describe the overall level of morning stiffness you have had from the time you wake up?

| 0 | 1 | 2 | 3 | 4 | ☒ | 6 | 7 | 8 | 9 | 10 |

none   very severe

Intensity of morning stiffness

6. How long does your morning stiffness last from the time you wake up?

| 0 | 1 | 2 | 3 | 4 | ☒ | 6 | 7 | 8 | 9 | 10 |

0 hr   2 or more hours

Duration of morning stiffness

BASDAI=4

Figure 6.30 Bath Ankylosing Spondylitis Disease Activity Index. In the example above, the BASDAI=4. The BASDAI is calculated by adding the mean of questions 5 and 6, to the sum of questions 1–4, the total figure is then divided by 5. AS, ankylosing spondylitis; BASDAI, Bath Ankylosing Spondylitis Disease Activity Index; NRS, numerical rating score. Adapted with permission from Garrett et al [75].

Assessment in SpondyloArthritis international Society core set for clinical record keeping

Domain	Application
1. Function	BASFI
2. Pain	NRS/VAS-last week-spine-at night-due to AS
	and NRS/VAS-last week-spine-due to AS
3. Spinal mobility	Chest expansion
	and modified Schober
	and occiput to wall
	and cervical rotation
	and (lateral spinal flexion or BASMI)
4. Patient global	NRS/VAS-global disease activity last week
5. Peripheral joints and entheses	Number of swollen joints (44 joint count)
	Validated enthesitis score, such as MASES,
	San Francisco and Berlin
6. Stiffness	NRS/VAS duration of morning stiffness-spine-last week
7. Acute phase reactants	Erythrocyte sedimentation rate
8. Fatigue	Fatigue question BASDAI

Figure 6.31 Assessment in SpondyloArthritis international Society core set for clinical record keeping. AS, ankylosing spondylitis; BASDAI, Bath Ankylosing Spondylitis Disease Activity Index; BASFI, Bath Ankylosing Spondylitis Functional Index; BASMI, Bath Ankylosing Spondylitis Metrology Index; MASES, Maastricht Ankylosing Spondylitis Enthesitis Score; NRS, numerical rating scale; VAS, visual analogue scale. Adapted with permission from van der Heijde et al [76].

Spondylitis Functional Index) is shown in Figure 6.32 and Figures 3.3–3.7 (see Chapter 3) showed how to measure spinal mobility [77]. BASDAI and BASFI should be assessed about every 3–6 months and spinal mobility about every 6–12 months, depending on the level of disease activity and progression of the disease. These instruments have also been used as outcome parameters in clinical trials. A more detailed description is given in the recently published ASAS handbook on the assessment of spondyloarthritis [78].

Bath Ankylosing Spondylitis Functional Index

Please indicate your level of ability with each of the following activities during the past week

All items scored on a 0–10 numerical rating scale* (0 = easy, 10 = impossible)

1. Putting on your socks or tights without help or aids (eg, sock aid)

2. Bending forward from the waist to pick up a pen from the floor without aid

3. Reaching up to a high shelf without help or aids (eg, a helping hand)

4. Getting up out of an armless dining room chair without using your hands or any other help

5. Getting up off the floor without help from lying on your back

6. Standing unsupported for 10 minutes without discomfort

7. Climbing 12–15 steps without using a handrail or walking aid (one foot at each step)

8. Looking over your shoulder without turning your body

9. Doing physically demanding activities (eg, physiotherapy, exercises, gardening or sports)

10. Doing a full days' activities, whether it be at home or at work

The BASFI is the mean of 10 item-scores completed on a numerical rating scale

Figure 6.32 Bath Ankylosing Spondylitis Functional Index. *A visual analogue scale (0–100) can also be used. BASFI, Bath Ankylosing Spondylitis Functional Index. Adapted with permission from Calin et al [77].

References

1   Braun J, van den Berg R, Baraliakos X, et al. 2010 update of the ASAS/EULAR recommendations for the management of ankylosing spondylitis. *Ann Rheum Dis*. 2011;70:896-904.

2   Anderson JJ, Baron G, van der Heijde D, Felson DT, Dougados M. Ankylosing spondylitis assessment group preliminary definition of short-term improvement in ankylosing spondylitis. *Arthritis Rheum*. 2001;44:1876-1886.

3   Song IH, Poddubnyy DA, Rudwaleit M, Sieper J. Benefits and risks of ankylosing spondylitis treatment with nonsteroidal anti-inflammatory drugs. *Arthritis Rheum*. 2008;58:929-938.

4   Amor B, Dougados M, Listrat V, et al. Are classification criteria for spondylarthropathy useful as diagnostic criteria? *Rev Rheum Engl Ed*. 1995;62:10-15.

5   Sieper J, Lenaerts J, Wollenhaupt J, et al; on Behalf of All INFAST Investigators. Efficacy and safety of infliximab plus naproxen versus naproxen alone in patients with early, active axial spondyloarthritis: results from the double-blind, placebo-controlled INFAST study, Part 1. *Ann Rheum Dis*. 2013 May 21. [Epub ahead of print].

6   Gossec L, Dougados M, Phillips C, et al; ASAS (ASsessment in AS international working group). Dissemination and evaluation of the ASAS/EULAR recommendations for the management of ankylosing spondylitis: results of a study among 1507 rheumatologists. *Ann Rheum Dis*. 2008;67:782-788.

7   Wanders A, Heijde Dv, Landewé R, et al. Nonsteroidal antiinflammatory drugs reduce radiographic progression in patients with ankylosing spondylitis: a randomized clinical trial. *Arthritis Rheum*. 2005;52:1756-1765.

8   Poddubnyy D, Rudwaleit M, Haibel H, et al. Effect of non-steroidal anti-inflammatory drugs on radiographic spinal progression in patients with axial spondyloarthritis: results from the German Spondyloarthritis Inception Cohort. *Ann Rheum Dis*. 2012;71:1616-1622.

9 Kroon F, Landewé R, Dougados M, van der Heijde D. Continuous NSAID use reverts the effects of inflammation on radiographic progression in patients with ankylosing spondylitis. *Ann Rheum Dis*. 2012;71:1623-1629.

10 Coxib and traditional NSAID Trialists' (CNT) Collaboration, Bhala N, Emberson J, et al. Vascular and upper gastrointestinal effects of non-steroidal anti-inflammatory drugs: meta-analyses of individual participant data from randomised trials. *Lancet*. 2013;382:769-779.

11 Bakland G, Gran JT, Nossent JC. Increased mortality in ankylosing spondylitis is related to disease activity. *Ann Rheum Dis*. 2011;70:1921-1925.

12 Haibel H, Fendler C, Listing J, Callhoff J, Braun J, Sieper J. Efficacy of oral prednisolone in active ankylosing spondylitis: results of a double-blind, randomised, placebo-controlled short-term trial. *Ann Rheum Dis*. 2013 May 16. [Epub ahead of print].

13 Braun J, Bollow M, Seyrekbasan F, et al. Computed tomography guided corticosteroid injection of the sacroiliac joint in patients with spondyloarthropathy with sacroiliitis: clinical outcome and followup by dynamic magnetic resonance imaging. *J Rheumatol*. 1996;23:659-664.

14 Haibel H, Rudwaleit M, Listing J, Sieper J. Open label trial of anakinra in active ankylosing spondylitis over 24 weeks. *Ann Rheum Dis*. 2005;64:296-298.

15 Haibel H, Rudwaleit M, Braun J, Sieper J. Six months open label trial of leflunomide in active ankylosing spondylitis. *Ann Rheum Dis*. 2005;64:124-126.

16 Haibel H, Brandt HC, Song IH, et al. No efficacy of subcutaneous methotrexate in active ankylosing spondylitis: a 16-week open-label trial. *Ann Rheum Dis*. 2007;66:419-421.

17 Braun J, Zochling J, Baraliakos X, et al. Efficacy of sulfasalazine in patients with inflammatory back pain due to undifferentiated spondyloarthritis and early ankylosing spondylitis: a multicentre randomised controlled trial. *Ann Rheum Dis*. 2006;65:1147-1153.

18 Dougados M, vam der Linden S, Leirisalo-Repo M, et al. Sulfasalazine in the treatment of spondylarthropathy. A randomized, multicenter, double-blind, placebo-controlled study. *Arthritis Rheum*. 1995;38:618-627.

19 Brandt J, Listing J, Sieper J, Rudwaleit M, van der Heijde D, Braun J. Development and preselection of criteria for short term improvement after anti-TNF alpha treatment in ankylosing spondylitis. *Ann Rheum Dis*. 2004;63:1438-1444.

20 Landewé R, Braun J, Deodhar A, et al. Efficacy of certolizumab pegol on signs and symptoms of axial spondyloarthritis including ankylosing spondylitis: 24-week results of a double-blind randomised placebo-controlled Phase 3 study. *Ann Rheum Dis*. 2013 Sep 6. [Epub ahead of print].

21 van der Heijde D, Dijkmans B, Geusens P, et al; Ankylosing Spondylitis Study for the Evaluation of Recombinant Infliximab Therapy Study Group. Efficacy and safety of infliximab in patients with ankylosing spondylitis: results of a randomized, placebo-controlled trial (ASSERT). *Arthritis Rheum*. 2005;52:582-591.

22 van der Heijde D, Kivitz A, Schiff MH, et al; ATLAS Study Group. Efficacy and safety of adalimumab in patients with ankylosing spondylitis: results of a multicenter, randomized, double-blind, placebo-controlled trial. *Arthritis Rheum*. 2006;54:2136-2146.

23 Davis JC, van der Heijde DM, Braun J, et al. Sustained durability and tolerability of etanercept in ankylosing spondylitis for 96 weeks. *Ann Rheum Dis*. 2005;64:1557-1562.

24 Braun J, Brandt J, Listing J, et al. Treatment of active ankylosing spondylitis with infliximab: a randomised controlled multicentre trial. *Lancet*. 2002;359:1187-1193.

25 Davis JC Jr, Van Der Heijde D, Braun J, et al; Enbrel Ankylosing Spondylitis Study Group. Recombinant human tumor necrosis factor receptor (etanercept) for treating ankylosing spondylitis: a randomized, controlled trial. *Arthritis Rheum*. 2003;48:3230-3236.

26 Inman RD, Davis JC Jr, Heijde Dv, et al. Efficacy and safety of golimumab in patients with ankylosing spondylitis: results of a randomized, double-blind, placebo-controlled, phase III trial. *Arthritis Rheum*. 2008;58:3402-3412.

27 van der Heijde D, Lie E, Kvien TK, et al. ASDAS, a highly discriminatory ASAS-endorsed disease activity score in patients with ankylosing spondylitis. *Ann Rheum Dis*. 2009;68:1811-1818.

28 Machado P, Landewé R, Lie E, et al; Assessment of SpondyloArthritis international Society. Ankylosing Spondylitis Disease Activity Score (ASDAS): defining cut-off values for disease activity states and improvement scores. *Ann Rheum Dis*. 2011;70:47-53.

29 Braun J, Landewé R, Hermann KG, et al; ASSERT Study Group. Major reduction in spinal inflammation in patients with ankylosing spondylitis after treatment with infliximab: results of a multicenter, randomized, double-blind, placebo-controlled magnetic resonance imaging study. *Arthritis Rheum*. 2006;54:1646-1652.

30 Rudwaleit M, Baraliakos X, Listing J, Brandt J, Sieper J, Braun J. Magnetic resonance imaging of the spine and the sacroiliac joints in ankylosing spondylitis and undifferentiated spondyloarthritis during treatment with etanercept. *Ann Rheum Dis*. 2005;64:1305-1310.

31 Lambert RG, Salonen D, Rahman P, et al. Adalimumab significantly reduces both spinal and sacroiliac joint inflammation in patients with ankylosing spondylitis: a multicenter, randomized, double-blind, placebo-controlled study. *Arthritis Rheum*. 2007;56:4005-4014.

32 Sieper J, Baraliakos X, Listing J, et al. Persistent reduction of spinal inflammation as assessed by magnetic resonance imaging in patients with ankylosing spondylitis after 2 yrs of treatment with the anti-tumour necrosis factor agent infliximab. *Rheumatology (Oxford)*. 2005;44:1525-1530.

33 Heiberg MS, Nordvåg BY, Mikkelsen K, et al. The comparative effectiveness of tumor necrosis factor-blocking agents in patients with rheumatoid arthritis and patients with ankylosing spondylitis: a six-month, longitudinal, observational, multicenter study. *Arthritis Rheum*. 2005;52:2506-2512.

34 Braun J, Deodhar A, Dijkmans B, et al; Ankylosing Spondylitis Study for the Evaluation of Recombinant Infliximab Therapy Study Group. Efficacy and safety of infliximab in patients with ankylosing spondylitis over a two-year period. *Arthritis Rheum*. 2008;59:1270-1278.

35 van der Heijde D, Schiff MH, Sieper J, et al; ATLAS Study Group. Adalimumab effectiveness for the treatment of ankylosing spondylitis is maintained for up to 2 years: long-term results from the ATLAS trial. *Ann Rheum Dis*. 2009;68:922-929.

36 Baraliakos X, Listing J, Fritz C, et al. Persistent clinical efficacy and safety of infliximab in ankylosing spondylitis after 8 years--early clinical response predicts long-term outcome. *Rheumatology (Oxford)*. 2011;50:1690-1699.

37 Braun J, Deodhar A, Inman RD, et al. Golimumab administered subcutaneously every 4 weeks in ankylosing spondylitis: 104-week results of the GO-RAISE study. *Ann Rheum Dis*. 2012;71:661-667.

38 Braun J, Baraliakos X, Listing J, et al. Persistent clinical efficacy and safety of anti-tumour necrosis factor alpha therapy with infliximab in patients with ankylosing spondylitis over 5 years: evidence for different types of response. *Ann Rheum Dis*. 2008;67:340-345.

39 van der Heijde D, Landewé R, Baraliakos X, et al; Ankylosing Spondylitis Study for the Evaluation of Recombinant Infliximab Therapy Study Group. Radiographic findings following two years of infliximab therapy in patients with ankylosing spondylitis. *Arthritis Rheum*. 2008;58:3063-3070.

40 van der Heijde D, Landewé R, Einstein S, et al. Radiographic progression of ankylosing spondylitis after up to two years of treatment with etanercept. *Arthritis Rheum*. 2008;58:1324-1331.

41 Maksymowych WP, Chiowchanwisawakit P, Clare T, Pedersen SJ, Østergaard M, Lambert RG. Inflammatory lesions of the spine on magnetic resonance imaging predict the development of new syndesmophytes in ankylosing spondylitis: evidence of a relationship between inflammation and new bone formation. *Arthritis Rheum*. 2009;60:93-102.

42 Brown MA, Kennedy LG, MacGregor AJ, et al. Susceptibility to ankylosing spondylitis in twins: the role of genes, HLA, and the environment. *Arthritis Rheum*. 1997;40:1823-1828.

43 Maksymowych WP, Morency N, Conner-Spady B, Lambert RG. Suppression of inflammation and effects on new bone formation in ankylosing spondylitis: evidence for a window of opportunity in disease modification. *Ann Rheum Dis*. 2013;72:23-28.

44 Baraliakos X, Haibel H, Listing J, Sieper J, Braun J. Continuous long-term anti-TNF therapy does not lead to an increase in the rate of new bone formation over 8 years in patients with ankylosing spondylitis. *Ann Rheum Dis.* 2013 Mar 27. [Epub ahead of print].

45 Haroon N, Inman RD, Learch TJ, et al. The Impact of TNF-inhibitors on radiographic progression in Ankylosing Spondylitis. *Arthritis Rheum.* 2013 Jul 1. [Epub ahead of print].

46 Braun J, Sieper J. What is the most important outcome parameter in ankylosing spondylitis? *Rheumatology (Oxford).* 2008;47:1738-1740.

47 Breban M, Ravaud P, Claudepierre P, et al; French Ankylosing Spondylitis Infliximab Network. Maintenance of infliximab treatment in ankylosing spondylitis: results of a one-year randomized controlled trial comparing systematic versus on-demand treatment. *Arthritis Rheum.* 2008;58:88-97.

48 Li EK, Griffith JF, Lee VW, Wang YX, Li TK, Lee KK, Tam LS. Short-term efficacy of combination methotrexate and infliximab in patients with ankylosing spondylitis: a clinical and magnetic resonance imaging correlation. *Rheumatology (Oxford).* 2008;47:1358-1363.

49 Vander Cruyssen B, Ribbens C, Boonen A, et al. The epidemiology of ankylosing spondylitis and the commencement of anti-TNF therapy in daily rheumatology practice. *Ann Rheum Dis.* 2007;66:1072-1077.

50 Braun J, Baraliakos X, Listing J, et al. Differences in the incidence of flares or new onset of inflammatory bowel diseases in patients with ankylosing spondylitis exposed to therapy with anti-tumor necrosis factor alpha agents. *Arthritis Rheum.* 2007;57:639-647.

51 Braun J, Baraliakos X, Listing J, Sieper J. Decreased incidence of anterior uveitis in patients with ankylosing spondylitis treated with the anti-tumor necrosis factor agents infliximab and etanercept. *Arthritis Rheum.* 2005;52:2447-2451.

52 Rudwaleit M, Rødevand E, Holck P, et al. Adalimumab effectively reduces the rate of anterior uveitis flares in patients with active ankylosing spondylitis: results of a prospective open-label study. *Ann Rheum Dis.* 2009;68:696-701.

53 Vincent FB, Morand EF, Murphy K, Mackay F, Mariette X, Marcelli C. Antidrug antibodies (ADAb) to tumour necrosis factor (TNF)-specific neutralising agents in chronic inflammatory diseases: a real issue, a clinical perspective. *Ann Rheum Dis.* 2013;72:165-178.

54 Rudwaleit M, Van den Bosch F, Kron M, Kary S, Kupper H. Effectiveness and safety of adalimumab in patients with ankylosing spondylitis or psoriatic arthritis and history of anti-tumor necrosis factor therapy. *Arthritis Res Ther.* 2010;12:R117.

55 Lie E, van der Heijde D, Uhlig T, et al. Effectiveness of switching between TNF inhibitors in ankylosing spondylitis: data from the NOR-DMARD register. *Ann Rheum Dis.* 2011;70:157-163.

56 Song IH, Heldmann F, Rudwaleit M, et al. Treatment of active ankylosing spondylitis with abatacept: an open-label, 24-week pilot study. *Ann Rheum Dis.* 2011;70:1108-1110.

57 Sieper J, Porter-Brown B, Thompson L, Harari O, Dougados M. Assessment of short-term symptomatic efficacy of tocilizumab in ankylosing spondylitis: results of randomised, placebo-controlled trials. *Ann Rheum Dis.* 2013 June 13. [Epub ahead of print].

58 Baeten D, Baraliakos X, Braun J, et al. Anti-interleukin-17A monoclonal antibody secukinumab in treatment of ankylosing spondylitis: a randomised, double-blind, placebo-controlled trial. *Lancet.* 2013;S0140-6736:61134-4.

59 Haibel H, Rudwaleit M, Listing J, et al. Efficacy of adalimumab in the treatment of axial spondylarthritis without radiographically defined sacroiliitis: results of a twelve-week randomized, double-blind, placebo-controlled trial followed by an open-label extension up to week fifty-two. *Arthritis Rheum.* 2008;58:1981-1991.

60 Sieper J, van der Heijde D, Dougados M, et al. Efficacy and safety of adalimumab in patients with non-radiographic axial spondyloarthritis: results of a randomised placebo-controlled trial (ABILITY-1). *Ann Rheum Dis.* 2013;72:815-822.

61 Dougados M, et al. Clinical and imaging efficacy of etanercept in early non-radiographic axial spondyloarthritis: a 12-week, randomized, double-blind, placebo-controlled trial. *Ann Rheum Dis.* 2013;72(Suppl):87.)

62 Barkham N, Keen HI, Coates LC, et al. Clinical and imaging efficacy of infliximab in HLA-B27-Positive patients with magnetic resonance imaging-determined early sacroiliitis. *Arthritis Rheum.* 2009;60:946-954.

63 Song IH, Hermann K, Haibel H, et al. Effects of etanercept versus sulfasalazine in early axial spondyloarthritis on active inflammatory lesions as detected by whole-body MRI (ESTHER): a 48-week randomised controlled trial. *Ann Rheum Dis.* 2011;70:590-596.

64 Song IH, Weiß A, Hermann KG, et al. Similar response rates in patients with ankylosing spondylitis and non-radiographic axial spondyloarthritis after 1 year of treatment with etanercept: results from the ESTHER trial. *Ann Rheum Dis.* 2013;72:823-825.

65 Song IH, Althoff CE, Haibel H, et al. Frequency and duration of drug-free remission after 1 year of treatment with etanercept versus sulfasalazine in early axial spondyloarthritis: 2 year data of the ESTHER trial. *Ann Rheum Dis.* 2012;71:1212-1215.

66 Haibel H, Heldmann F, Braun J, Listing J, Kupper H, Sieper J. Long-term efficacy of adalimumab after drug withdrawal and retreatment in patients with active non-radiographically evident axial spondyloarthritis who experience a flare. *Arthritis Rheum.* 2013;65:2211-2213.

67 Sieper J, Lenaerts J, Wollenhaupt J, et al; on Behalf of All INFAST Investigators. Maintenance of biologic-free remission with naproxen or no treatment in patients with early, active axial spondyloarthritis: results from a 6-month, randomised, open-label follow-up study, INFAST Part 2. *Ann Rheum Dis.* 2013 Jun 5. [Epub ahead of print].

68 Horneff G, Fitter S, Foeldvari I, et al. Double-blind, placebo-controlled randomized trial with adalimumab for treatment of juvenile onset ankylosing spondylitis (JoAS): significant short term improvement. *Arthritis Res Ther.* 2012;14:R230.

69 van der Heijde D, Sieper J, Maksymowych WP, et al; Assessment of SpondyloArthritis international Society. 2010 Update of the international ASAS recommendations for the use of anti-TNF agents in patients with axial spondyloarthritis. *Ann Rheum Dis.* 2011;70:905-908.

70 Keat A, Barkham N, Bhalla A, et al; BSR Standards, Guidelines and Audit Working group. BSR guidelines for prescribing TNF-alpha blockers in adults with ankylosing spondylitis. Report of a working party of the British Society for Rheumatology. *Rheumatology (Oxford).* 2005;44:939-947.

71 Maksymowych WP, Gladman D, Rahman P, et al; Canadian Rheumatology Association/ Spondyloarthritis Research Consortium of Canada. The Canadian Rheumatology Association/ Spondyloarthritis Research Consortium of Canada treatment recommendations for the management of spondyloarthritis: a national multidisciplinary stakeholder project. *J Rheumatol.* 2007;34:2273-2284.

72 Spondylitis Association of America. Physician Resources - Guidelines for the Use of TNF-a Therapy. www.spondylitis.org/physician_resources/guidelines.aspx.

73 Rudwaleit M, Listing J, Brandt J, Braun J, Sieper J. Prediction of a major clinical response (BASDAI 50) to tumour necrosis factor alpha blockers in ankylosing spondylitis. *Ann Rheum Dis.* 2004;63:665-670.

74 Rudwaleit M, Schwarzlose S, Hilgert ES, Listing J, Braun J, Sieper J. MRI in predicting a major clinical response to anti-tumour necrosis factor treatment in ankylosing spondylitis. *Ann Rheum Dis.* 2008;67:1276-1281.

75 Garrett S, Jenkinson T, Kennedy LG, Whitelock H, Gaisford P, Calin A. A new approach to defining disease status in ankylosing spondylitis: the Bath Ankylosing Spondylitis Disease Activity Index. *J Rheumatol.* 1994;21:2286-2291.

76 van der Heijde D, Calin A, Dougados M, Khan MA, van der Linden S, Bellamy N. Selection of instruments in the core set for DC-ART, SMARD, physical therapy, and clinical record keeping in ankylosing spondylitis. Progress report of the ASAS Working Group. Assessments in Ankylosing Spondylitis. *J Rheumatol.* 1999;26:951-954.

77 Calin A, Garrett S, Whitelock H, et al. A new approach to defining functional ability in ankylosing spondylitis: the development of the Bath Ankylosing Spondylitis Functional Index. *J Rheumatol.* 1994;21:2281-2285.

78 Sieper J, Rudwaleit M, Baraliakos X, et al. The Assessment of SpondyloArthritis international Society (ASAS) handbook: a guide to assess spondyloarthritis. *Ann Rheum Dis.* 2009;68 Suppl 2:ii1-44.